Zainichi Koreans and Mental Health

Using a qualitative, interview-based approach, Kim investigates how conflicting identities and social marginalization affect the mental health of members of the ethnic Korean minority living in Japan.

So-called "Zainichi" Koreans living in Japan have a higher suicide rate than native Japanese, or than any other ethnic group within Japan, a country which has one of the highest suicide rates in the world. Considering themselves neither truly Korean nor wholly Japanese, they are mainly descendants of immigrants who came to Japan during the colonial period in the late 19th and early 20th centuries. Kim explores the challenges facing these individuals, including the dilemmas of ethnic education, the discrimination against them by mainstream society, and the consequent impacts on their mental health.

An insightful read both for scholars of Japanese culture and society and for anthropologists and sociologists with an interest in the effects of marginalization on ethnic minority citizens more broadly.

Taeyoung, Kim, also known as Izawa, Yasuki, is a Professor in the Department of Sociology at Toyo University, Japan. He is a third-generation "Zainichi" Korean naturalized in Japan.

Routledge Contemporary Japan Series

For more information about this series, please visit: www.routledge.com/
Routledge-Contemporary-Japan-Series/book-series/SE0002

Zainichi Koreans and Mental Health

Psychiatric Problem in Japanese Korean Minorities, Their Social Background and Life Story

Taeyoung Kim

Routledge
Taylor & Francis Group

LONDON AND NEW YORK

First published 2022
by Routledge
2 Park Square, Milton Park, Abingdon, Oxon OX14 4RN

and by Routledge
605 Third Avenue, New York, NY 10158

Routledge is an imprint of the Taylor & Francis Group, an Informa business

© 2022 Taeyoung Kim

British Library Cataloguing-in-Publication Data
A catalogue record for this book is available from the British Library

Library of Congress Cataloguing-in-Publication Data
A catalog record has been requested for this book

ISBN: 9781032010823 (hbk)
ISBN: 9781032010830 (pbk)
ISBN: 9781003177050 (ebk)

DOI: 10.4324/9781003177050

Typeset in Galliard
by KnowledgeWorks Global Ltd.

Contents

List of figures

List of tables

Introduction

For minorities, society is very stressful. Minorities constantly experience disrespect, discrimination, exclusion, and ostracism in society based on attributes such as ethnicity, gender, place of birth, sexuality, and "disability." This is not an essentialism "because he/she is a minority," but is caused by the social structure in which anyone is susceptible if treated that way. As a result of such stress, minorities experience various forms of suffering in life. And, as stress continues to build up over time, persons experiencing such stress are considered to be at high "risk" for the onset of mental disorders.

Stress can be easily handled as a subjective matter. For persons who are sensitive and easily affected by pressure, such pressure can lead to physical and/or mental disorders. On the other hand, some persons are not concerned about the same pressure, or redirect the pressure into positive energy. Consequently, stress tends to greatly depend on a person's individual responsibility. This also applies in the cases involving social minorities. The various feeling of unreasonableness and illogic the person experiences are easily cast aside as "you think too much," or "you're being paranoid."

Zainichi Koreans are one minority. This document focuses on the position of Zainichi Koreans in Japanese society, their experiences due to such position, the kind of stress they felt, and social environmental factors leading to mental disorder.

One result of these reasons is the high suicide rate of Zainichi Koreans. According to data which will be presented later, the suicide rate of Zainichi Koreans is higher than those of Japanese and other foreigners (although asserting so may be misleading). In addition, the issue of mental disorder can be found on the path leading to suicide. Psychiatrist, Youji Kurokawa, who died in 2008, noted that "seeing Zainichi North/South Koreans in daily psychiatric care is not uncommon."

In actual conditions however, studies which address the issue of Zainichi Koreans and mental disorders have not been actively carried out. In the same book, Dr. Kurokawa also stated that "there are very few papers which address mental disorder issues among Zainichi North/South Koreans."

There are some reasons for this. While mental disorders themselves carry some stigma, some "consideration" may be given to the hesitance to connect this issue with Zainichi Koreans as it may promote a sense of discrimination. On the other hand, it can be said that Zainichi Korean themselves view this issue as taboo, due to a strong sense of stigma connected with mental disorder within Zainichi Korean society. Although there are some people who are Zainichi Koreans and who have mental disorder, they are placed in the fringes of Zainichi Korean society which is already on the fringes of Japanese society. I wonder if, within the issue of Zainichi Koreans and mental disorder, the history, experiences, and memory of Zainichi Koreans are simply condensed and attributed to the fact that they are Zainichi Koreans.

As of the end of June 2019, approximately 2.83 million foreigners live in Japan. This is approximately 2% of total population in Japan. In 1999, the number of foreign residents in Japan exceeded 1.51 million persons, approximately 1.2% of total population. Between 1999 and 2019, the number of foreign residents temporarily decreased due to the Lehman Brothers bankruptcy and the Great East Japan Earthquake, but continued to increase after 2013. While the degree varies by area, seeing people with a different skin or hair color in cities is no longer uncommon. Communities of "new comer" foreigners have also been established in many areas.

On the other hand, the birthrate in Japan has continued to decline. Total fertility rate, which shows the number of children a woman bears in her lifetime, was 1.36 in 2019. At this rate, the population in Japan is said to decrease to one half in 80 years. The productive age population, from 15 to 64 years old, was 68.4% of the total population in 1999 but decreased to 59.5% in 2019. As estimated by the Ministry of Health and Welfare, a decrease to 54.6% by 2050 is predicted, and a severe labor shortage in the future is of concern. To compensate, it is easy to imagine a resurgence of the idea of "foreigners as a labor force." Japanese society has definitely made progress toward a multiethnic society.

Up to now, we have aimed for the "establishment of identity." Each person has sought to answer the question, "who am I?" and strives to become someone. Some people search for ways to identify themselves as members of a country, while others seek to identify themselves with their "race" or "ethnicity." However, within the identification of one's own existence, factors such as "essence," "natural," and "absolute" began to weaken after the 80s. Although not really essential, these factors have been historically and socially constructed. They are fluid and unstable, and efforts to view them "relatively" have been attempted.

Zainichi Koreans make up approximately 11% of the total foreign residents in Japan. In late 80s, Koreans occupied nearly 90% of all foreigners, and "Zainichi" (meaning foreigners who "live in Japan") was once used to signify "Zainichi Koreans." However, the proportion of Zainichi Koreans has continued to decrease each year.

Moreover, the conditions of the Zainichi Korean society have also greatly changed. The core of Zainichi Koreans has shifted from first generation Koreans who were born in Korea, to second, third, fourth, fifth and even sixth generation Japan-born Koreans. Their social standing in Japanese society, the workings of Zainichi Korean society, and the position of their identity have also greatly changed. Some view the condition as a "loss of ethnicity," while others view it as "diversification." On the other hand, the viewpoint of seeking new possibilities from within the chaos can also be seen.

The issue of identity faced by Zainichi Koreans can be viewed as an original issue for Zainichi Koreans, but it can also apply to other races and ethnic groups. From a wider viewpoint, the issue is universal, shared by anyone who lives in modern society. In this book, I would like to consider the modern identity issues faced by Zainichi Koreans, especially by their statements and activities.

1 History and actual condition of Zainichi Koreans

Up to this point, the term "Zainichi Korean" has been used without providing a specific definition. Who are "Zainichi Koreans"? At the beginning of this book, the term "Zainichi Korean" was used as the "general term for persons with roots in the Korean Peninsula who were directly or indirectly affected by Japan's colonial domination over the Korean Peninsula and who moved to Japan." In modern society, determining to what extent should various persons be included (or would like to be included) within the scope of "Zainichi Korean," and who should not be included (or would like to not be included), has become difficult. Here, "Zainichi Korean" include persons of South Korean, North Korean, persons with Japanese, or other citizenship.

Attributes of Zainichi Koreans have also become more complicated, such as persons who were born from parents of North/South Korean, Japanese, and/ or other nationalities, referred to as "double" (or "half"). Within that meaning, self-definition as "Zainichi Korean" as an objective indicator (nationality, etc.) has become difficult and has become closer to the subjective indicator that "I am a Zainichi Korean," or "I am one of those people who are called Zainichi Korean." In other words, "Zainichi Koreans" are ethnic minorities with roots in the Korean Peninsula who have been directly and indirectly affected by Japan's colonial domination over the Korean Peninsula, and then moved to Japan. They are also comprised of persons with various attributes and are subject to disrespect and discriminatory treatment even in modern society.

As Table 1.1 shows, there was a time in Japan where "foreigners in Japan" used to refer to "Zainichi Koreans." However, the proportion gradually decreased, and in modern times, "Zainichi Koreans" becomes one of many foreigners. Among these the "Number of North/South Koreans" who entered Japan after the 1980s, called "newcomer Koreans," are also included in "Zainichi Koreans." Among the "Number of North/South Koreans," the number of "special permanent residents" almost coincides with the number of Zainichi Koreans. "Special permanent resident" is a residence status regulated by the "Special Act on the Immigration Control of Inter Alia, Those Who Have Lost Japanese Nationality Pursuant to the Treaty of Peace with Japan," under the Japanese law that came into effect on November 1, 1991. Persons targeted by this Act include "persons who have lost Japanese Nationality Pursuant to a Treaty of Peace," or "a

DOI: 10.4324/9781003177050-1

Table 1.1 Changes in the number of North/South Korean nationals in Japan (prepared based on "Changes in the Number of Foreign Residents" (previously "Changes in the Number of Registered Foreign Nationals") by the Ministry of Justice)

Year	Number of foreign residents in Japan	Number of North/South Koreans	Composition rate (%)
1978	766,894	659,025	85.9
1979	774,505	662,561	85.5
1980	782,910	664,536	84.9
1981	792,946	667,325	84.2
1982	802,477	669,854	83.5
1983	817,129	674,581	82.6
1984	840,885	687,135	81.7
1985	850,612	683,313	80.3
1986	867,237	677,959	78.2
1987	884,025	676,982	76.6
1988	941,005	677,140	72.0
1989	984,455	681,838	69.3
1990	1,075,317	687,940	64.0
1991	1,218,891	693,050	56.9
1992	1,281,644	688,144	53.7
1993	1,320,748	682,276	51.7
1994	1,354,011	676,793	50.0
1995	1,362,371	666,376	48.9
1996	1,415,136	657,149	46.4
1997	1,482,707	645,373	43.5
1998	1,512,116	638,828	42.2
1999	1,556,113	636,548	40.9
2000	1,686,444	635,269	37.7
2001	1,778,462	632,405	35.6
2002	1,851,758	625,422	33.8
2003	1,915,030	613,791	32.1
2004	1,974,747	607,419	30.8
2005	2,011,555	598,687	29.8
2006	2,084,919	598,219	28.7
2007	2,069,065	582,754	28.2
2008	2,144,682	580,760	27.1
2009	2,125,571	571,598	26.9
2010	2,087,261	560,799	26.9
2011	2,047,349	542,182	26.5
2012	2,033,656	530,048	26.1
2013	2,066,445	519,740	25.2
2014	2,121,831	501,230	23.6
2015	2,232,189	491,711	22.0
2016	2,382,822	485,557	20.4
2017	2,561,848	481,522	18.8
2018	2,731,093	479,193	17.5

Table 1.2 Changes in the number of special permanent residents and percentage of North/South Koreans (prepared based on "Changes in the Number of Foreign Residents" by the Ministry of Justice)

Year	North/South Koreans	Special permanent residents	Percentage of North/ South Koreans (%)
1999	636,548	517,787	81.3
2000	635,269	507,429	79.9
2001	632,405	495,986	78.4
2002	625,422	485,180	77.6
2003	613,791	471,756	76.9
2004	607,419	461,460	76.0
2005	598,687	447,805	74.8
2006	598,219	438,974	73.4
2007	582,754	430,229	73.8
2008	580,760	420,305	72.4
2009	571,598	409,565	71.7
2010	560,799	399,106	71.2
2011	542,182	389,085	71.8
2012	530,048	381,364	71.9
2013	519,740	373,221	71.8
2014	501,230	358,409	71.5
2015	491,711	348,626	70.9
2016	485,557	338,950	71.8
2017	481,522	329,822	68.5
2018	479,193	321,416	67.1

descendant of a person who has lost Japanese Nationality Pursuant to a Treaty of Peace," and specifically North/South Koreans and Taiwanese who lost Japanese nationality pursuant to the San Francisco Peace Treaty that came into effect on April 28, 1952. Among special permanent residents, persons with nationalities other than North/South Korean comprise 1% of the total. In other words, almost all special permanent residents are North/South Koreans. Consequently, the number of special permanent residents is considered to indicate the number of Zainichi Koreans.

However, as shown in Table 1.2, the percentage of special permanent residents who are Korean-registered is steadily decreasing. This is because the elderly are dying and the number of people who acquire Japanese nationality is increasing. One reason for the decrease in the North/South Korean population is the aging and death of first-generation Zainichi Koreans. A second reason is an increase in the number of persons obtaining Japanese citizenship. Table 1.3 shows the changes in the number of North/South Koreans who obtained Japanese citizenship. A total of 380,303 persons obtained Japanese citizenship between 1952 and 2019.

A third reason is the change in citizenship inheritance by children of an international marriage due to revision of the Japanese Nationality Act in 1985. Citizenship can now be based on the nationality of either the father or mother, drastically reducing the number of persons who choose to inherit North/South Korean citizenship. Due to these reasons, the Zainichi Korean population has decreased.

Table 1.3 Changes in the number of North/South Koreans who obtained Japanese citizenship (prepared based on "Changes in the Number of Applicants for Naturalization Permission" by the Ministry of Justice)

Year	Number of people	Year	Number of people	Year	Number of people	Year	Number of people	Year	Number of people
1952	232	1967	3,391	1982	6,521	1997	9,678	2012	5,581
1953	1,326	1968	3,194	1983	5,532	1998	9,561	2013	4,331
1954	2,435	1969	1,889	1984	4,608	1999	10,059	2014	4,744
1955	2,434	1970	4,646	1985	5,040	2000	9,842	2015	5,247
1956	2,290	1971	2,874	1986	5,110	2001	10,295	2016	5,434
1957	2,737	1972	4,983	1987	4,882	2002	9,188	2017	5,631
1958	2,246	1973	5,769	1988	4,595	2003	11,778	2018	4,357
1959	2,737	1974	3,973	1989	4,759	2004	11,031	2019	4,360
1960	3,763	1975	6,323	1990	5,216	2005	9,689	Total	380,303
1961	2,710	1976	3,951	1991	5,665	2006	8,531		
1962	3,222	1977	4,261	1992	7,244	2007	8,546		
1963	3,558	1978	5,362	1993	7,697	2008	7,412		
1964	4,632	1979	4,701	1994	8,244	2009	7,637		
1965	3,438	1980	5,987	1995	10,327	2010	6,668		
1966	3,816	1981	6,829	1996	9,898	2011	5,656		

One may think that, as the Zainichi Korean population continues to decrease and nears zero, issues related to the discrimination of Zainichi Koreans within Japanese society would also end. However, such thing will not happen. Almost 100 years have passed since Zainichi Koreans first started to come to Japan, and discrimination by Japanese against Zainichi Koreans has continued to be passed down. In recent years, hate speech targeting Zainichi Koreans has become widespread. During street demonstrations and on the Internet, slogans such as "Expel all Koreans from Japan, good or bad!" "Eliminate all the Koreans!" are shouted out loud. On the other hand, some forms of discrimination are difficult to see directly. There are issues of microaggression and aversive racism against Zainichi Koreans.

1.1 Zainichi Koreans and social distance

A questionnaire on hate speech and historical awareness was jointly carried out by Zainichi Korean youth organizations in 2013 (respondents: 1,014 university students in Tokyo, Osaka, Kyoto, and Fukuoka). Awareness of "social distance" toward Zainichi Koreans was surveyed.

The "social distance scale" is a measure of psychological affinity one has toward individuals and groups. Generally, the social distance between persons who are recognized as members of the ingroup is short, however, the distance increases toward members of the outgroup. Bogardus prepared a scale to measure social distance based on whether an individual accepts or rejects a member of another group.

Bogardus identified 60 items, such as "marriage," "feelings regarding the person marrying one's brother or sister," and "becoming best friends" (Bogardus, 1933). For example, questions for each case, such as "if your brother or sister were to marry a Korean, would you approve or disapprove?" "If a Korean wanted to be your friend, would you approve or disapprove?" When the answer is "I would approve," it is judged as "high receptivity" or "favorable." When the answer is "I would disapprove," it is judged as "high rejectivity" or "unfavorable." Through questions such as these, awareness to specific groups can be determined. In Japan, there are few studies that utilize this "social distance." As a representative example, there is one study by Hiroshi Wagatsuma and Toshinao Yoneyama (1967). In this study, ten questions were asked regarding persons of "English, French, German, American, Italian, Indian, Russian, Thai, Ethnic Chinese, Indonesian, Filipino, Korean ethnic group, black, white mixed race, or black mixed race descent," namely "If a ... becomes your close friend," "If a ... becomes close friends with your family," "If a ... goes on a trip with you," "If a ... lives in Japan," "If a ... goes to school with you or your children," "If a ... lives next door to you," "If a ... is naturalized in Japan and becomes a Japanese citizen," "If a ... enters a bath or pool with you," "If a ... sleeps in the same room at a inn as you," "If a ... were to marry your brother, sister or child," and the responses were analyzed. In a survey by myself and others in 2013, five items from among the ten items described above, namely 1) "If a ... lives in Japan," 2) "If a ... wants to become your friend," 3) "If a ... will live next door to you," 4) "If a ... goes on a trip with you," 5) "If your brother, sister or relative will marry a ..." were used.

Figure 1.1 shows the results of social distance awareness toward "North/South Koreans." As expected, as social distance decreases, "approve" decreases and "disapprove" increases. Moreover, "disapprove" was higher than "approve" for "marriage."

As previously described, social distance measures the receptivity or rejectivity toward an outgroup. According to the results, as the distance from Zainichi Koreans decreases, receptivity was observed to decrease and rejectivity increases. In addition, regarding questions of "marriage," the tendency was shown to be noticeably higher for "disapprove" than to "approve."

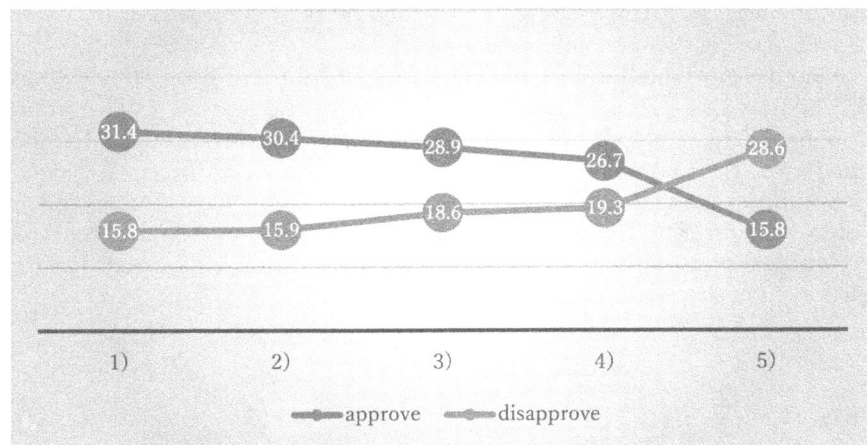

Figure 1.1 Social distance awareness toward North/South Koreans (%).

Table 1.4 "Job Conditions of Zainichi Koreans" (1955)

By job category	Number of people	Ratio by job category (%)
Agriculture	10,156	1.8
Manufacturing	24,573	4.6
Commerce	31,023	5.8
Transportation	5,266	0.9
Civil Engineering/ Construction	19,991	3.7
Food and Beverage	5,157	0.9
Gaming	7,207	1.3
Marine transport	612	–
Trade	163	–
Mining	–	–
Fisheries	801	–
Intellectual workers	7,237	1.3
Daytime workers	35,585	6.6
Unemployed	13,269	2.4
Jobless	328,624	61.3
Other	46,084	8.5
Total	535,803	100.0

(Source: Shinozaki, 1955. "History Textbook - Zainichi Korean History" Preparation Committee (2013)

According to "History Textbook - Zainichi Korean History," Preparation Committee (2013), Japanese workers from coal and other mines, as well as factories, were mobilized to the battle lines during the Korean War. Many Zainichi Koreans were also drafted or forced to work to fill deficiencies in support of the wartime industry. After the war however, demobilized Japanese returned to their work and Zainichi Koreans were discharged from their workplaces. After the war, things went back to normal for the Japanese, but for Zainichi Koreans, they no longer had steady jobs and were worse off than the Japanese, and many had a real life of "poverty and wandering."

According to Table 1.4, the total population of Zainichi Koreans in 1952 was 535,803 persons. Among these, 61% were jobless, and daytime workers comprised the largest proportion of employed people at 6.6%. Although the job category is listed as "commerce," most work involved waste material collection or working at eating establishments in stores such as the military barracks and or selling makkori (Korean homemade fermented sake) and horumonyaki (beef and pork grilled meat) on the black market ("History Textbook - Zainichi Korean History" Preparation Committee (2013)).

2 "Zainichi" Korean and mental disorders

2.1 Studies on Zainichi Koreans and mental disorders

There are few studies on Zainichi Koreans and mental disorders. Here, the works of three psychiatrists are introduced.

At the time of his study, Kazue Ohashi (1980) pointed out that Zainichi Koreans are "Japan's largest minority group" and "marginal persons" forced to live while internalizing the centrality and marginality of Japanese society and at the same time trying to understand this internally. "When cultural differences, ethnicity, and history result in actual clinical problems, these problems mainly occur in the psychoneurosis field. In addition to minor cases within the psychological area, such cultural differences, ethnicity, and history may also trigger early phase onset of a disorder and affect the timing of social rehabilitation."

Youji Kurokawa (2006) noted that "seeing Zainichi North/South Koreans in daily psychiatric care is not uncommon," but "there are very few papers addressing mental disorder issues specifically among Zainichi North/South Koreans." The paper by Ohashi is "the only paper where the author focuses on Zainichi Koreans and Korean persons."

Moreover, regarding reasons for the difficulty in addressing this issue and developing approaches within this background, Kurokawa mentioned 1) deep discrimination that looks down Orientals, which was created by the "Out of Asia and Into Europe" Meiji ideology, 2) Zainichi North/South Koreans are not recognized as "foreigners" (Zainichi North/South Koreans are recognized by Japanese only when targeted for discrimination), 3) issues such as "discrimination and prejudice" are overly politicized and considered taboo, and have, in a way, become "holy ground," and 4) the viewpoint of disease based on the traditional psychiatric medicine is dominant, and social factors involved in mental disorders, etc., are often ignored.

Kurokawa also mentions 1) psychopathology of mental disorders observed in Zainichi North/South Koreans (issues such as identity formation, onset preparation condition, onset condition, psychogenesis, clinical picture formation, and chronicity), 2) issues regarding treatment of Zainichi North/South Koreans (development of cases, issues of compulsory hospitalization, patient/healer relationship, aid organization, discrimination structure underlying psychiatric care),

DOI: 10.4324/9781003177050-2

and 3) other psychological and social problems (discrimination, poverty, cultural conflict, etc.) affecting Zainichi North/South Koreans, as issues in psychiatric medicine and care.

In addition, he points out that "many levels are involved in the regulating of the existence of Zainichi North/South Koreans, such as historical, political, cultural, socio-economically, and psychological levels. These causes and the resulting "discrimination structure" are considered to be important. The "Zainichi North/South Koreans issue" did not exist as a priori, but occurred within the interaction with Japanese people, and likely became an issue of the Japanese people."

What brings a definitive effect in the formation of the Zainichi North/South Korean identity is the existence of a "discrimination structure" that dominates life and one's entire existence. Three types of identity are thought to be formed with this background, namely 1) Marginal Identity: existence like a "half-Japanese," where one does not identify with either Japanese or Korean, 2) Counter Identity: formed to overcome conflict or struggle in opposition to the Japanese identity, and when connected with misconduct or crime is called a Negative Identity, and, 3) As-If Identity: in cases where one lives by superficially adopting a Japanese lifestyle but hides one's true ethnicity in order to escape discrimination and exclusion, even though not completely assimilated to Japanese. Kurokawa states, "Regardless of which identity is achieved, if there is not a safety valve within the Japanese society, it will lead to crisis."

Generally, identity conflict is considered to be a characteristic pathology in adolescence. However, in cases of Zainichi North/South Koreans, it should be noted that this sometimes appears in early old age. Japanese society does not allow a Zainichi North/South Korean to accept him/herself as is or to assimilate to Japanese society. The "general configuration and social structure constantly drives them to insanity." In addition, from the position of traditional psychiatric medicine, Kurokawa considers social factors, such as discrimination and prejudice, poverty, and cultural friction, which regulate the existence of Zainichi North/South Koreans, as patoplastisch (pathoplastic) and provozier-end (incentive) within the "mental disorder structure."

Next, according to Kim Jangsu (2001), in cases of Zainichi Koreans, in addition to identity crisis coming from the position of a minority in Japanese society, conflict between North/South Korean culture and Japanese culture is thought to greatly influence occurrence, clinical picture, and disease progression. Kim pointed out that there are not only individual genetic components, but also environmental factors, in other words, social, cultural, and family factors, and these have a stronger effect.

Moreover, the rate of treatment and consultation for Zainichi Koreans is higher than that for Japanese at Dr. Kim's clinic because there are many Korean residents in the area and he himself uses his own ethnic name.

Dr. Kim states that Zainichi Koreans, first of all, "vacillate their existence between Japan, North/South Korea." Every time the political relationship between Japan, North Korea, or South Korea becomes tense, Zainichi Koreans become caught in the middle, and have no choice but to be concerned about the relationship between these countries. Second, although Zainichi Koreans consider "North/South Korea as their birth parent and Japan as their adopted parent," they are in the painful condition of being fostered against their will and not receiving enough love from their foster parent. Third, Zainichi Koreans have a "difficult-to-see existence, or an invisible existence." Population-wise, although their numbers are not so low, the existence of Zainichi Koreans is difficult to be seen by Japanese people. There are also Japanese people who try not to see Zainichi Koreans, and Korean residents who try not to be seen. Fourth, Zainichi Koreans are also viewed as "People who speak Japanese." This group is not considered Japanese, but they are not North/South Korean because they speak Japanese. This designation is accompanied with a strong nuance, where people underestimate themselves and are without identity. This mainly applies to second and third generation Zainichi Koreans.

Being a minority in Japanese society and the conflict between North/South Korean culture and Japanese culture in society is considered to greatly influence onset, the clinical picture, and progression. In cases of "Zainichi," not only are there individual genetic components, but also environmental factors. In other words, social, cultural, and family factors have a stronger effect. As general characteristics of mental disorders of Zainichi Koreans, the following points can be raised: 1) in many cases, the patient experiences economic difficulties, 2) the background of disease is complicated, 3) details of the disease are complicated, 4) strong aversion to clinical psychiatry, 5) strong inclination to non-scientific treatment, and 6) strong stigma of mental disorders.

The following points are raised as common characteristics according multiple cases: 1) experience of being bullied due to ethnic discrimination, 2) abrupt change in life due to accident/earthquake disaster, 3) raised in a dysfunctional household, and 4) suffering from adult children syndrome (AC).

Kim indicates that, according to various cases, in addition to experiencing bullying in early childhood, many Zainichi Korean patients with mental disorder were raised in such dysfunctional households and as a result have AC-like personalities. Kim calls Zainichi Koreans who experience identity crisis along with AC-like personality tendencies, as "Zainichi syndrome" patients. Mental disorder occurs as one's personality is distorted in a distorted environment. On the other hand, while some people with "Zainichi syndrome," have aspects that can be easily identified as mental disorder, others show a different side. One form is where they try to overcome and recover from Zainichi syndrome, but when they fail, they revert to so-called anti-social activities. Another form is they work hard to apply themselves to the recovery process, and to some degree, are able to display a certain amount of success. To do this, effort by the person is needed. Warmth and cooperation from others and a certain amount of good luck are also important conditions. For these reasons the social status of people with Zainichi syndrome significantly differs depending on the person, and as this difference increases, the social status as a minority appears.

2.2 Discrimination and stress based on a survey of actual conditions

According to Selye, stress is a condition characterized by a unique syndrome consisting of various changes induced in biological tissue in a non-specific manner (Selye, 1956-1988). "Non-specific" is defined as what can "occur in any case." When a state of tension develops within an individual due to an internal stimulation that can be a physical or mental burden, event, or condition, or due to an external stimulation that can cause stress, such stimulations are referred to as stressors. Stressors can be physio-chemical, physical, psychological, environmental, or social (Katou, 2001). Selye defined environmental and social stressors as "social/cultural stressors." For example, he indicated that "cross-cultural stress" is felt by persons who are easily considered as unfavorable intruders by the receiving residents, such as immigrants and foreigner workers. These new visitors can easily suffer from a lack of friendship or social contact because they are expected to follow not only the customs and food (of the land) but also the general sense of life, which is vastly different than their own. However, it is wrong to view "stress=bad influence." While "bad stress" can adversely affect a person when in excess, "good stress" is said to help a person to grow.

Generally, when an individual is exposed to an external environmental factor (stressor), he changes his vital environment to adapt to it. This is referred to as the stress response. Stress response is called a "two-edged sword." It is a biological defense function in case of an emergency, while at the same time, it can cause various ailments when prolonged.

Stress can be acute stress or chronic stress. "Acute" occurs when an event or a critical situation suddenly occurs. "Chronic" is sustained and continuous stress. Stress experienced by Zainichi Koreans as discussed here is chronic stress, which is felt daily as a Zainichi Korean.

A survey on the actual condition of discrimination of Zainichi Korean youth regarding hate speech and Internet use (hereinafter referred to as "Survey of Actual Condition of Discrimination of Zainichi Korean Youth") targeting 203 Zainichi Koreans (18–39 years old, of South Korean, North Korean, and Japanese nationalities) living in Tokyo, Osaka, Hyogo, and other areas was carried out jointly with the Zainichi Korean youth organization from June 2013 to March 2014. In this survey, Zainichi Korean youth were asked to describe their daily life experiences. From the written descriptions, the experiences of Zainichi Korean youth in their daily life are introduced here.

"The parents of my Japanese partner opposed because I am Zainichi."
"I got married to a Japanese concealing that I am a Zainichi."
"I hid the fact that I am a Zainichi Korean from my Japanese husband, but when he found out, our marital relationship suddenly cooled."
"Relatives on the Japanese side look on our relationship with disapproval."
"We eloped because my spouse's parents strongly opposed our marriage."

"Because it's difficult to pronounce my name in South/North Korean, others
gave me pretty simplified nickname."
"I was called "Chon-Koh""
"When I told a friend that I am Zainichi Korean, he said "Go back to your
own country.""
"I was forced to use my real name."
"People take every opportunity to treat me like an enemy"

If a public official or public agency/company makes a discriminatory speech in
public for example, it would be a problem. But speech and actions between individuals are hard to expose or turn into an issue.

> What hurt the most was not being understood. "Why you are in Japan?"
> "Why can't you speak Korean?" Even if I explain, they aren't listening.
> There is no intention to understand. If I criticize Japan's colonial domina-
> tion, they would say, "why not go back to South Korea." [32-year-old man,
> South Korean nationality]
>
> When I was a third or fourth grade elementary school student, my best
> friend's grandmother wouldn't let me enter their house. The friend said "I
> don't really understand, but my grandma says you cannot come in because
> you are a child of Korea." I went home but didn't understand what hap-
> pened. After many years, I thought "Oh, that was discrimination." [28-year-
> old woman, Japanese nationality]
>
> When I told a person whom I trusted that I am Zainichi, the person
> said "You're you. Our relationship won't change" but I felt like she didn't
> understood. The friend, whom I thought understood me, wrote something
> discriminatory against China, so I thought I couldn't trust her. I don't
> think I can tell others who I am because I worry if "they hate Zainichi,"
> or that they only make a face like they understand. [21-year-old woman,
> Japanese nationality]
>
> If I don't tell those who become my friends that I am Zainichi, I feel like
> I am hiding something. It's difficult when an acquaintance doesn't know I
> am Zainichi and the topic of the election comes up and asks "who did you
> vote for in the election?" When I was in college and my roommate told her
> father that I am "Zainichi" (just told him the facts in passing), he opposed
> us being roommates. (After that though, no particular problem developed,
> and we still lived together). Another time, when I stopped near the imperial
> palace in Hayama to look at the map, I was asked to show ID, and when
> the person found out I was "Zainichi", he asked for my cell phone number.
> [34-year-old woman, South Korean nationality]
>
> When I wanted to rent a house, I was strongly asked to use a common
> name (I protested and didn't sign the contract). I used a common name
> to hide my nationality and transferred to a Japanese junior high school.
> However, on the day of opening ceremony, a classmate who heard about
> me from a teacher told me to meet behind the school building, and beat

me saying, "you're Korean, aren't you?" When I was talking with a friend in Korean, someone all of a sudden spoke abusively saying "You Korean bastard". [33-year-old man, South Korean nationality]

I knew there were conditions for a foreigner to become a full-time teacher (in Japan). When I took the Japanese Teaching Staff Examination, there wasn't a place to write one's nationality on the application, so I asked when nationality would be considered. I was told to write "South Korean nationality" on a piece of paper and attach it to the application. I do not know if this is discrimination or not, but I think not having a column to describe one's nationality is wrong, even though there are conditions regarding nationality. [23-year-old woman, South Korean nationality]

After I was hired prior to graduation, I was called to the company and asked to give a Japanese name. They said, "identifying yourself with your real name is your own choice, but if the client finds out (you are Zainichi), you might be discriminated against. This can cause problems for other employees." [37-year-old man, South Korean nationality]

I applied for home school when I was a freshman in high school, but was denied because the contents taught in Korean school are different. It did not change even when my parents called. [20-year-old woman, North Korean nationality]

When I was a senior in high school (I was going to Korean school), I wanted to take a university entrance examination for selected candidates, but I was told that students from the Korean school were not eligible and I couldn't take the exam after all. When I asked the reason, I was given an ambiguous answer that I wasn't attending a high school. From the following year, it seems that students after me could take the exam and enter (that university). [29-year-old woman, South Korean nationality]

When I was a junior high school student, my family was moving into a house, but the owner refused to let us move in after he found out we were Zainichi Korean. [34-year-old man, North Korean nationality]

In high school, we were told in art class to make a clay model of a person's face. I heard a classmate near me say "it looks like a Korean," referring to a statue with slanted eyes and a distorted face. I felt uncomfortable, but kept silent and didn't do anything. [19-year-old woman, Japanese nationality]

Since "Japan's annexation of the Korean Peninsula," the history of Zainichi Koreans in Japan has already passed more than 100 years. However, discrimination and disrespect toward "Zainichi" still remains in Japanese society today. Zainichi Koreans live their daily lives with such discrimination and disrespect.

2.3 Zainichi Koreans and suicide rate

Up to this point, one thing in particular represents the stress issues faced by Zainichi Koreans – the rate of suicide. Suicide is said to be closely related to mental disorders. According to the WHO (World Health Organization), 90% of people who kill themselves in high-income countries have mental disorders, and persons with more than two mental disorders have a significantly higher risk of suicide (WHO, 2014).

Factors in the onset of mental disorders are generally said to be a complicated mix of genetic, temperament, and socio-environmental factors. In the case of minorities who are likely to experience social discrimination and mental disorders, it is important to consider socio-environmental factors. Minorities receive tangible and intangible stress because they are a minority. How does this affect the mental and psychological condition of minorities, and lead to mental disorder? These points must be considered. While many studies on this subject have been accumulated in Europe and US, few have been carried out in Japan.

The suicide rate in Japan by nationality is shown in Figure 2.1 and prepared based on "Vital Statistics in Japan," by the Health, Labour and Welfare Ministry, and the Suicide Statistics and Reference Chart issued by the Office for Suicide Prevention Policy, Cabinet Office, Community Safety Planning Division, Community Safety Bureau, and National Police Agency.

According to the chart, the suicide rate of South/North Koreans is higher than for Japanese (entire population) and other foreigners. These figures are considered to indicate the difficult condition Zainichi Koreans face, as seen up to now.

However, setting the suicide rate of "South/North Koreans" as the "suicide rate of Zainichi Koreans" is misleading. Since there is currently no "suicide rate according to individual resident status" in the statistics, the number of

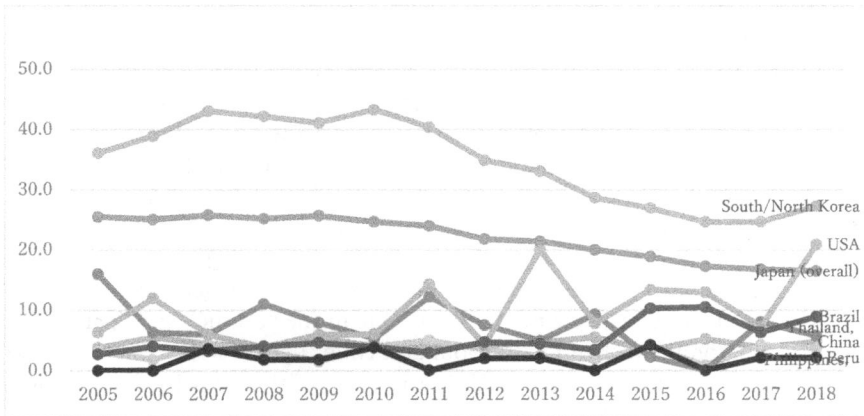

Figure 2.1 Suicide rate in Japan by nationality (number per 100,000 persons).

Note: Prepared based on "Vital Statistics in Japan," Health, Labour and Welfare Ministry, suicide victims based on the Suicide Statistics and Reference Chart, Office for Suicide Prevention Policy, Cabinet Office, Community Safety Planning Division, Community Safety Bureau, National Police Agency and "Change in Number of Foreign Residents," Ministry of Justice.

Zainichi Koreans and the number of so-called "newcomer Koreans" among these "South/North Koreans" (roughly the number persons whose resident status is "special permanent resident") is not known. Among these "South/North Koreans," both of Zainichi Koreans and newcomer Koreans are included.

However, even in such circumstances, the high suicide rate among South/North Koreans is considered to be influenced by the condition of Zainichi Koreans. One reason is that if only "newcomer Koreans" are abstracted and separated from the suicide rate, the number is almost the same as the suicide rate for other foreigners. Another reason is that, as indicated by WHO for example, the rate of death by suicide is still higher in minorities and in persons who experience discrimination, and discrimination to persons of lower status occurs within the population group even today. In addition, this is regionally specific and systematic. This is caused by continued experience of life events with high stress, such as loss of freedom, rejection, stigma, and violence, which lead to suicide-related actions (WHO, 2014).

As previously shown, Zainichi Koreans live with various stress in Japanese society. The suicide rate of Zainichi Koreans (or person with North/South Korean nationality) can be considered to be a direct demonstration of this fact.

When shown this statistical data, Japanese so-called "online right-wingers" become critical saying "emphasizing victim awareness again?" "South Korea also has a high suicide rate! Isn't it ethnicity?" In response to such opinions, the suicide rate between South Koreans and Zainichi Koreans is compared. Suicide rates between Zainichi Koreans, South Korean, and Japan overall are compared in Figure 2.2.

According to the chart, the gap between rates has decreased in recent years, but the rate for Zainichi Koreans is still higher than that for South Koreans. In other words, this high suicide rate for Zainichi Koreans is influenced by socio-environmental factors, not "ethnicity."

This situation of Zainichi Koreans is also reflected in personal experience.

Mr. K is a second generation of Zainichi Korean who engaged in regional activities in Zainichi Korean residential areas for many years. Within ten years, he lost four close friends, including his own brother, to suicide. All his friends who committed suicide were Zainichi Koreans. The following interview was held with Mr. K by e-mail.

> Looking at my brother, he was the first son and second generation Zainichi Korean. I think he had a more difficult life in the "ethnic" and "paternalistic" environment, than I as the youngest child. Let me write about my close friends who killed themselves. This is in order of their deaths. By the way, I was also born in 1957.
>
> Friend A: Woman, Born in 1957. Second generation Korean. The woman was tired due to her daughter's eating disorder. After working for a student movement, the woman went to Korea for a year to confirm her own identity. She was central person in a cultural movement that focused on ethnic culture festivals. She jumped off a building.

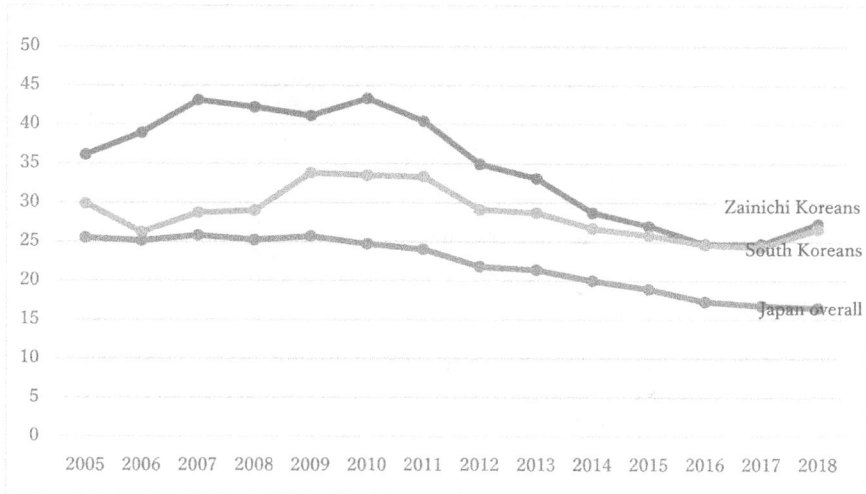

Figure 2.2 Suicide rate of Zainichi Koreans, South Koreans, and Japan overall.

Note: Prepared based on "Vital Statistics in Japan," Health, Labour and Welfare Ministry, and suicide victims based on the Suicide Statistics and Reference Chart, Office for Suicide Prevention Policy, Cabinet Office, Community Safety Planning Division, Community Safety Bureau, National Police Agency, "Change in Number of Foreign Residents," Ministry of Justice, and OECD Data: Suicide rates (https://data.oecd.org/healthstat/suicide-rates.htm)

Friend B: Woman, Born in 1957. Second generation Korean. She was working for a Zainichi youth movement since her youth and fought for the Cultural movement and the release of Zainichi women. Her daughter committed suicide when she was in law school. Several years later, the woman killed herself too. She jumped off a building Friend.

C: Man Born in 1957. Has actively engaged in ethnic activities since high school.

At first, he couldn't go to South Korea, a country of dictatorship, but eventually he could go, and participated in a tour that addressed the issue of comfort women and the military. He committed suicide(?) while in South Korea. He was found dead in the ocean.

The three people mentioned above were very good friends of mine. They can be called my best friends since my 20's. Friend A called me 10 days before committing suicide and said she "wanted me to introduce her to a psychiatrist." I was so worried about her but could only introduce her to a psychiatrist. It has become a mental scar.

Friend D: Born in 1959. Man. Third generation Korean. He was involved in an ethnic movement as a student. After graduating, he managed a home school with his brother. However, with the onset depression, he put a charcoal barbeque in his car and committed suicide by carbon monoxide poisoning.

Brother: Born in 1952. Second generation Korean. He was the first son and bore much responsibility in a "paternalistic" environment. He established a successful business, but invested in real estate during the bubble era, resulting in much debt. In the process, he developed a brain disease and became physically-disabled. He continued to manage a factory, but eventually the company failed. Several weeks before he committed suicide, he called each of his brothers and sisters to talk. Among siblings, I was the closest to him. He gave me music CDs, expensive brandy, etc. I said, "you're not thinking about doing something strange, aren't you?" But I never imagined he would commit suicide. Is that because I viewed him as a "strong" brother since childhood? He hung himself and died.

On paper, these experiences may sound dull, but each one of them, especially the deaths of Friends A and C, and my brother left permanent damage on me. Every year, on the day of my brother's death, I cannot sleep all night until the morning, even now.

And, he added, "Losing 5 close people in 10 years by suicide is not normal. Japanese people cannot imagine this."

3 Compound discrimination and mental disorder/suicide in Zainichi Korean women

Korean women in Japan are subject to multiple discrimination. It is discrimination against Koreans and discrimination against women.

With the problem of "compound discrimination" in the background, Zainichi Korean women have a difficult time living. The term "compound discrimination" was coined by Chizuko Ueno, and can be described as follows.

> An individual lives as a social being in many contexts simultaneously. A weak person facing discrimination in one context can be a strong person in another context. There are many cases where a person facing discrimination, also experiences multiple discrimination at the same time as a socially weak person. However, the relationship between these various forms of discrimination are sometimes complex within the identity of the person himself/herself, and results in conflict.
>
> (Ueno, 1996, 203–204)

Yuriko Moto states the following.

> Minority women, whether in the "women" category or marginalized while belonging to a group, are in a position where they cannot be seen and their voice cannot be heard. Consideration of compound discrimination can be a useful tool in illuminating and analyzing the situation, can encourage society to take appropriate action and empower women as a minority.
>
> (Moto, 2018, 14)

Jung Yeonghae indicated contradictions in the national liberation movement among first-generation Zainichi Korean.

> Traditionally, the national liberation movement developed by first generation "Zainichi Koreans" included a major contradiction. Because with few exceptions, most of the supporters were men and while outwardly advocating ethnic liberation, suppressed women and children in the background.

DOI: 10.4324/9781003177050-3

The distressing life of first generation "harumoni" (mothers) was created by their own husbands, and at the same time, by Japan's imperialism.

(Jung, 1996, 10)

Jung applied the words of Yang Yong Ja and described discrimination issues faced by this Zainichi Korean "ethnic" group.

They were firmly bound by the Confucian system. In addition to house-work and raising children, there was pressure to respect ancestors through festivals, and show devotion to one's parents-in-law. Women who do not get married were viewed as "disabled persons who are not human." Persons advocating release by ethnic liberation excluded them from "humans" with the same tongue. After women get married, they must keep getting preg-nant until they give birth to a boy, then work as laborers in the household industry. Furthermore, women were strictly forbidden to have the same social standing and intellectual level as men - "women should not become involved in politics and men's talk." In reality, wives were slaves to their husbands.

(Jung, 1996, 11; Yang, 1985)

Under such conditions, it is not uncommon for Zainichi Korean women to be driven to mental disorder and suicide. Suicide rate for Japan overall, Koreans in Japan, by men and women, is shown in Figure 3.1.

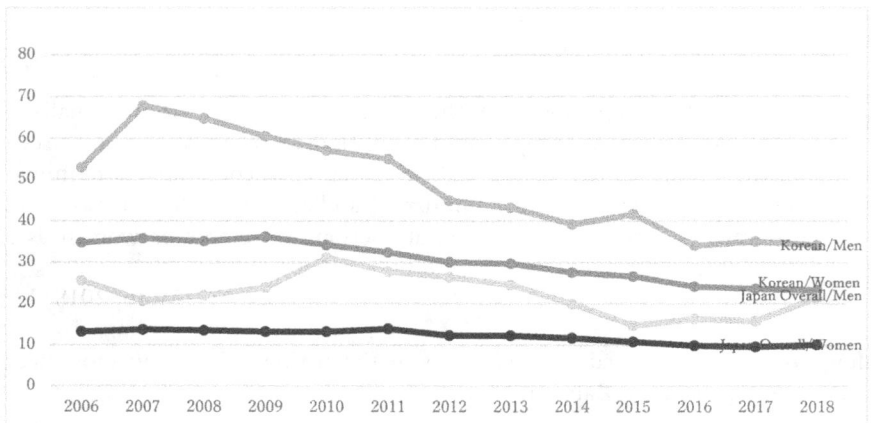

Figure 3.1 Suicide rate of "Japan overall," Koreans in Japan, and ratio of men and women.

Note: Prepared based on "Vital Statistics in Japan," Health, Labour and Welfare Ministry, suicide victims based on the Suicide Statistics and Reference Chart, Office for Suicide Prevention Policy, Cabinet Office, Community Safety Planning Division, Community Safety Bureau, National Police Agency and "Change in Number of Foreign Residents," Ministry of Justice.

Suicide rate in the order of high to low was "Korean/Men," "Japan Overall/ Men," "Korean/Women," and "Japan Overall/Women," and the tendency was consistent. In 2007, when the suicide rate for "Korean/Men" was the highest, the gap between "Japan Overall/Men" was 1.9 times. In 2010, when the suicide rate of "Korean/Women" was the highest, the gap between "Japan Overall/ Women" was 2.4 times.

Moreover, the average suicide rate from 2006 to 2018 in "Korean/Men" was 48.5 persons and "Japan Overall/Men" was 30.3 persons. The gap between these groups was 1.6 times. "Korean/Women" was 22.3 persons, "Japan Overall/Women" was 12.1 persons, and the gap was 1.8 times.

Accordingly, it was clear that suicide rate of Koreans in Japan was consistently higher than that for Japan Overall. In addition, Zainichi Korean women, who are the theme of this article, also had a consistently higher suicide rate.

Up to now, the overall picture of the severe condition of Zainichi Koreans and Zainichi Korean women has been viewed through statistical resources. From here, the actual image of Zainichi Korean women and their difficulties in life are specifically described in detail according to an interview survey carried out in May 2019.

For the survey in this section, Ms. S, a second-generation Zainichi Korean woman (70 years old) who was employed at a welfare center in the Kansai region, was interviewed. Survey contents included the details and conditions of Zainichi Korean women cared for by Ms. S and who suffered mental disorders.

The purpose of this study was verbally explained to Ms. S in advance, and that she could discontinue the study if she felt she was unable to cooperate, did not have to answer a question if she did not want to, if consent is obtained, her responses would be recorded, the data would only be used for purposes of the study. When talking about cases, the persons would be referred to as "Ms. A, Ms. B," so the interviewer would not know the personal name of the patient, and when this is published as thesis, the personal name of the individuals would not be specified in the description, and then consent was obtained. Moreover, in this article, important episodes were revised and designed so individuals were not specified.

Case 1: Ms. A

Did you know many people have taken wives from Korea? Approximately 40 years ago, Korea was poor. The poorest country in the world, it was shortly after the Korean War had ended. The Treaty on Basic Relations between Japan and Republic of Korea was established in 1965. At the time, I was very poor, and was not making much money in Japan. So I started to go back to my hometown, and go back and forth, bringing many brides from South Korea. One of the brides was my neighbor, from Gyeongsangnam-do. Probably people who can't find a Japanese wife and can't get married would find a wife from South Korea. Have you heard about it?

One of these men, my brother's classmate, thought he wouldn't be able to get married, so his father went to South Korea and asked his acquaintances. Then, she came. About the person who came, as expected, if she were rich, she wouldn't have come to Japan, during that time. So I think she was pretty poor over there, too. When she came over, she even thought that she wouldn't get along with her husband, but wouldn't admit it because they do not understand the same language and mutually misunderstood each other. Family life didn't go well because they couldn't communicate due to the language, but they thought they would be able to understand each other one day, they lived as best they could. They had a child, my brother is a friend of the husband, so he asked me "to name the baby," so I named the girl. After that, a boy was born, so they had a girl and a boy.

There was a problem with the husband's father. Ultimately, I think "Zainichi" came to Japan after the war. They came in the late 1930s or early 1940s. So, their customs are those of South Korea around that time. From about 1965, South Korea began to change, they started to have various ways of thinking. But many fathers still had the way of thinking of 30 years ago, even after 1965, they would have the mindset of the 30s. Those fathers thought that when the wife was expecting a girl, normally in Japan, she would go back to own mother's house to give birth. But she had nowhere to go. Her mother had already passed away. So she gave birth at a maternity home with the father and son, and my brother was there. When they came home, the father said to a person in neighborhood, "I don't have rice to feed a wife who gives birth to a girl."

You have to feed something to the wife when she comes back from the maternity home, hospital, don't you? He didn't. If her husband tried to feed her, his father would get angry. The father was strange man, and the wife had a real hard time with him. Her husband tried to feed her something to eat secretly, but she became a little crazy. About the wife. The wife suffered a mental disorder after that.

The son (husband) told her to go home once, because she was lonely in Japan, without friends, and her parents are not here. He told her to go back and rest a little, so she went back, but over there, she was forced back to Japan. Even when she went back, the family said she was sent to Japan to reduce the number of mouths to feed. It wouldn't happen today, but it was nearly 50 years ago. She had so many problems, so she came back to Japan, but her illness became worse. She continued to get worse, and then she became paranoid, but her husband did not take her to the hospital. Then she was paranoid and eventually jumped in front of a train.

She jumped in front of the train, and then a few years later, when the daughter became a high school student, the daughter also jumped in front of the train because she couldn't live with the father. A few years later, the son hung himself. Three people committed suicide. Since they died, about 10 years have passed. The people around them started to have more money and a better life style, maybe for the children. They may have wondered why only their family doesn't get better. As children, they were ok, but when they grew up, both the girl and boy also suffered depression.

That woman, the mother, died 20 years ago. After that, the father, daughter, and son lived together, but the son died about 10 years ago, or maybe more. So no one became happy, people in the neighborhood said "the mother took all of them." But the original cause was the husband's father.

The father pressured them. I was surprised when I heard that, and the neighbors are saying the same thing. I heard from a person in the neighborhood that the father was saying "I have no rice to feed a wife who gives birth to a girl." He told that to Japanese in the neighborhood. Surely for a Japanese person, everyone was surprised.

It's strange to say that now, people in Korea won't say that anymore. But that was the thinking when they came to Japan. That's why it is stopped there. Korea has been changing though. "Zainichi" is something that one continues to think about. Korea has been changing, but people who came to Japan have not changed. Even Buddhist memorial services as well. People in Korea do not have such memorial services. The Zainichi keep the memorial services which they have paid for, retaining their identity as Koreans. They seek identity there. They are not aware of it, but it is in there, like something Koreans are supposed to do.

They are arguing with each other. Families where the first generation is still alive, practice Buddhist memorial services. Families where the first generation has died, no longer practice it. It is a common trend. Are they arguing about Buddhist memorial services? Everyone was arguing and it became very serious. When I said I can't go because I have to work as a welfare manager, the mother pressured me very much. So work is more important, then? But for people in the first generation, it is different. This is like telling the daughter-in-law "You should take off from work for the Buddhist memorial service." If she says "I can't," she would be severely criticized. Poor thing.

Anyway, the way of thinking by the first-generation parents is totally different from the second generation. There was pressure from the parents. Parents in Korea do not have that much power, but Zainichi do. It's okay to do that to their own sons, but they also pressure their daughter-in-laws too. The daughter-in-laws must have had a hard time. So, it's easy for the presumptuous people to live, and while it's better in Japan, it's a difficult time for the poor. I think it is the same, regardless of the generation, but in today's world, very presumptuous people continue living. So, all the people who suffer mental disorders are quiet people. I don't think it is genetic, the way of thinking is passed down to the next generation, producing the same thinking across generations.

Case 2: Ms. B

A young girl developed schizophrenia. She was second generation, living in my neighborhood and she failed in love. She was smart, witty, but failed in love. Schizophrenia is often said to appear during puberty, right? She had sisters, and now that I think about it, I think the mother was also a little strange. She was the third daughter of three girls, and the youngest was a boy, the three girls had a younger brother, the last child. The brother hanged himself in the house. And the third girl is now about 60 years old. In her late 60s.

She was an outpatient at a mental hospital, diagnosed with schizophrenia. I heard she fell in love when she was about 20 years old. Of course the other person said he didn't want to marry a Korean, and her family also opposed at the time.

The other person was Japanese. The other side opposed, but opposition from first-generation Zainichi is unusual, isn't it? Opposition from both sides, eventually led to her being diagnosed with schizophrenia, and that was a problem. Once she started to talk, she wouldn't stop. When we are caught, sometimes she catches her "old sister," she says her ancestors are Russian. I don't think her face looks Russian, but she talks like she is a descendant of a rich, noble Russian family. Well, at least I think so. Even now she regularly goes to the psychiatric department, and receives welfare service there. A woman there has been taking care of her, though.

I also heard that the brother was living in a housing-development complex, and committed suicide. It was quite a while ago, maybe when he was in 30s. Maybe I can find it out if I ask her, but I don't think I can. No, I haven't asked. Her health is not good, and sometimes I help her too. Her husband collects cans, so I told him he could have ours too and I collect them for him. One time, she was admitted to the hospital due to brain stroke, I wonder if her condition is poor. You've heard that this may occur due to failed love, haven't you? So, I've heard Ms. C situation is just like that.

Case 3: Ms. C

Ms. C is an older lady, she has something… It's not Alzheimer's… She uses this facility now. She's in her 70s. But from her early 70s, she had problems with a neighbor, and I heard she was screaming. But she has calmed down since she came here. I don't know anything. I heard she screams loudly at her neighbor. So it's not normal dementia. It must be a mental disorder. I wonder if she visits the hospital.

She came to Japan to work, and her children are in Jeju, Korea. She came here to work, but ran into trouble for overstaying her visa. Her cousin, who is 10 years older than she, introduced her to his friend, an older Japanese man. The deal was, if she took care of the older Japanese man, he would marry her. It's a strange story, but not uncommon. Then, I don't know from when, she was taking care of the old man. The man was old, older than 90 years. So, it's difficult because he's old. Ms. C was about 63, at that time.

Now, the husband is in the hospital. She was taking care of him for all this time. But now, the Japanese man is in the hospital and cannot be released. Ms. C lives in his house now. Someone has to take care of her now, and that is her cousin. The cousin is 85 years old. The cousin is 10 years older than she, and only watches the house, and doesn't take care of her at night. Her diapers are not changed. She is brought to this facility with soiled diapers. So, what can I say? To survive.

The community general support center contacts us. For she is in a pretty bad condition, causing problems due to screaming at her neighbors. Now, she can only speak in Korean. She can't speak any Japanese. Maybe even in Korean, her speech is gibberish. I have no idea. Maybe she has schizophrenia. Maybe she is delusional and has auditory hallucinations or flashbacks. But she has seen a psychiatric physician.

Ms. C got married 22 or 23 years ago, today she is about 77 years old. So, she overstayed her visa when she was in her 50s, and her acquaintance arranged her marriage. Then she married an older man. Her husband is now 90, born in 1923 (Showa 3). Someone who was born in 1922 (Showa 2) is 91 years old. Or 92? He owned a vegetable store and was very successful. Ms. C married him after his wife died.

Ms. C had no problems, but was very quiet. Too quiet. Every time I brought the neighborhood new bulletin (kairanban) to her house, she was so shy, maybe she couldn't speak Japanese well. And, she was very pretty. She started to act strangely these past 5 or 6 years.

Her husband suffered a stroke. He suffered a stroke one time over 10 years ago and was paralyzed on one side. As a complication, now he is in the hospital due to a fractured right hip. He is paralyzed on the right side. He used his wife like his servant. So she was his maid. I'm sure that was the cause. Ms. C's anger was suppressed for these past 20 years. I really think so.

It seemed like she didn't have any friends, and every morning at 6 o'clock she would talk with the Korean grandma on the corner of the street in Korean for many hours, looking miserable. I kept thinking they should have gone to the cafe and have a cup of tea, but they just talked quietly at such a lonely place. Just to survive, she got married when she overstayed her visa.

So, it was because of suppression. Discrimination and suppression are the same, though. The person I previously talked about, she also experienced suppression from her father-in-law, right? She was also a quiet person, the daughter-in-law. Yes, she was also a quiet person, but could not bear the suppression by herself. Discrimination and suppression, that's it. So this is not normal social life, but in one aspect, she also was helped. But many people who overstay their visas in Japan are in the same situation. And many of them have fake marriages in order to stay in Japan. All humans have hard time just to survive. I think Zainichi Koreans face discriminations in Japanese society, they have hard time living well.

3.1 Discussion

3.1.1 *Confucian philosophy and discrimination against women*

Korea on the Korean Peninsula is a society with a stronger Confucian sense of thinking than Japan. In the world of first- and second-generation Zainichi, Confucian thinking and standards are strongly reflected in life. However, such thinking has changed in their "mother country," Korea.

Recently, the concept of the traditional family in Korea has significantly changed along with societal changes. Many Koreans wish to live independently as they grow old, rather than depending on their children. If a couple cannot resolve differences, they can divorce, and the idea of not having children and living satisfying lives by themselves has spread. An only child can be a son or a daughter, and marriage is not necessary if the person does not want to. Such changes in values have occurred along with economic development since the 1960s, and such changes have accelerated in recent years.

(Kim, Lee, 2007, 119)

The Confucian viewpoint has already changed in the "mother country." But for many Zainichi Koreans who immigrated to Japan (regardless of whether forced or voluntary), the traditional Confucian values and customs still remain intact. In the discussion of ethnicity and nationalism that exist in "enclaves" or "long-distance areas" that are separated from the "mother country," there exists an ethnic enclave theory and a long-distance nationalism theory.

Portes defined an "ethnic enclave" as "a group of immigrants concentrated in a specific spatial location and who organize an original ethnic market and various corporations to provide services to the general residents" (Portes, 1981, 290–291).

And, for this ethnic enclave to exist, two obvious requirements must be satisfied. First, ethnic entrepreneurs employ persons of the same ethnic group. Second, the ethnic enclave must be spatially limited from the main economy of the host society, so that it can function as an internal labor market. For example, connection by ethnic language, cultural knowledge, a social network with the mother country, as well as specific human capital skills are important. Marketability is high only in the internal labor market as defined by the ethnic enclave. (Xie & Gough, 2011)

Moreover, Benedict Anderson advocates the thinking of long-distance nationalism. This is a series of claims and practices of identity that connect people who live in various geographical points to a specific region which they view as the "home" of their ancestors. Similar to other forms of nationalism, nationalists who are separated far away believe that there is a country which is comprised of people who share a common history, identity, and region. On the other hand, it differs from other forms of nationalism in terms of the relationship between members of the country and those of the territory (Schiller, 2005).

However, both ethnic enclaves and long-distance nationalism mainly focus on the economic and political aspects, and there is hardly any description of culture and ethnicity of people who live in the "enclave" or "long-distance area." In other words, if Zainichi Koreans lived in their mother country, they could be released from some of the restrictions because the traditional culture has changed over time. However, since they live in an "enclave" or "long-distance area" where the collective resident district or community of "Zainichi", especially Zainichi Koreans, still retain the traditional culture and values, and its viewpoint and life customs, their lives remain suppressed, without release from the restrictions.

3.1.2 *Composition of a patriarch system and social construct of a dysfunctional family*

Lee and DeVos, et al. carried out an interview survey on Zainichi Koreans in the late 1970s, and described the "disdain by wives toward their husbands" as a characteristic of the Zainichi Korean household. Zainichi Koreans in Japanese society face discriminatory treatment in daily life and in important of aspects of their life, such as employment and marriage. As a result of such discriminatory treatment, men are especially excluded from the opportunities to gain stable work appropriate to their ability and qualifications. While Japanese men of the same age can obtain stable work, Zainichi Korean men are employed in insecure and unstable work conditions.

In the "Zainichi" families where Confucian values remain strong, a patriarchal system where the father retains the authority as the head of the family is ensured. On the other hand, this also means that the father is expected to fulfill the role and responsibilities of the head of the family. In addition to providing emotional and normative support of the family, this role also includes guaranteeing economic stability for the family. Through such responsibilities, fathers gain respect as the head of the family. However, many Zainichi Korean men cannot accomplish this. As a result, the wives and children think, "fathers of all the other families provide a steady income and a stable life for their families, why can't our father do so?" which leads to the evaluation that "he is helpless." These fathers are aware of such evaluation by their family, and their dignity is hurt. With a double meaning, they are disdained as Zainichi Koreans in society and as a "failed authority as the head of the family" at home. The fathers try to vent such stress through alcohol and violence to the family, leading to dysfunction in the family. In addition to or in spite of this, women "have to continue to 'forgive' these men who suppress them saying 'Father isn't being domineering, he couldn't help but to get drunk and act violently because he is lonely.'" (Jung, 1996, 10).

3.1.3 *Intergenerational trauma*

The collective experience of shared historical trauma experienced by social minorities, such as native tribes, when combined with the collective memory, sustained social and cultural disadvantage, and actions that increase the vulnerability for transmission and expression of the trauma effect between generations, is called "Intergenerational trauma" or "transgenerational trauma." Trauma can lead an individual to further stressors, and increases the reaction to these stressors.

The link between generations is observed in some behavioral disorders related to stress or trauma experience (depression, anxiety disorder, post-traumatic stress disorder, substance abuse disorders, etc.). Experience, evaluation, coping strategy, and chronic state of stressors, controllability, and predictability, which depend on variables such as age, gender, and childhood, can affect a person's vulnerability to pathologies (Bombay, 2014).

In the case of Ms. A, as a mother under Confucian values, she suffered onset of mental disorder and was driven to the point of suicide, and so were her two children. In the case of Ms. B, her background is not clear, but her brother also committed suicide. These facts indicate that the condition of Zainichi Koreans, their families, women, and children was traumatic and transmitted.

Up to this point, compound discrimination issues in Zainichi Korean women, which lead to mental disorders and suicide issues, have been identified through statistical resources and interview survey results. Zainichi Korean women bear much stress in Japanese society due to discriminatory treatment as Zainichi Koreans and discriminatory treatment as women, and this becomes a cause leading to mental disorders and suicide.

It became clear that persons of Korean nationality in Japan have a significantly higher suicide rate than "Japan Overall" and persons of other nationalities. The rate is also higher than that in South Korea, the "original country." In addition, when comparing men and women, the suicide rate was found to be higher in the order of "Korean/Men," "Japan Overall/Men," "Korean/Women," and "Japan Overall/Women." Suicide rate of both men and women of Korean nationality is higher than that for Japanese as a whole. From these facts, the amount and depth of stress experienced by Zainichi Korean women can be understood.

Next, the life history of three Zainichi Korean women was recounted by a second-generation Zainichi Korean woman who worked as a caregiver at a welfare center frequented by many Zainichi Korean women. Those three people lived with Confucian values in the Zainichi Korean world, and received discriminatory treatment as Zainichi Koreans. This led to mental disorder and suicide, not only for themselves but also their children who were driven to commit suicide as a result of the trauma link between generations. Such difficult facts could also be identified.

Racial factors often include appearance, but in the case of Zainichi Koreans, they do not look very different from Japanese. As for culture, they have already been assimilated into Japanese society. Another fact is that the onset factors of mental disorders of this minority group are difficult to visualize. Zainichi Korean women do not receive discriminatory treatment due to cultural difference, but receive discriminatory treatment because they are Korean. Furthermore, Zainichi Korean women are "a minority within a minority," relegated to a greater peripheral position even among Zainichi Koreans due to compound discrimination. Of course, the history and experience of Zainichi Korean women are original, differing from those by Zainichi Korean men. Onset of mental disorders and the background driving some to commit suicide are the result of their original background and circumstances. Ignoring "Zainichi Korean's…" is to hide one's originality and produces violence. This study and its implementation were carried out with constant awareness that we personally should not hide the problems of minority women including Zainichi Korean women, nor become perpetrators of violence.

4 The life stories of four Zainichi Koreans with mental disorders

Here, the life histories of four persons identified as "Zainichi Korean" and who suffer from mental disorder are introduced. These people were allowed to read the manuscript in advance and provided consent for inclusion.

4.1 Life story of Mr. A

4.1.1 *Condition at the time of the interview*

Currently, Mr. A is certified with a Grade 3 disability. For the past two years, he has worked as an accountant assistant at a company, based on the Act on Employment Promotion of Persons with Disabilities. According to Mr. A, he currently suffers from the "after effects of schizophrenia." He says "Now, my body cannot sleep without sleep medicine. If I don't take it, I will be up all night." Actually, Mr. A continued to talk about his own experiences and thoughts during the interview and could understand his own experiences and thoughts objectively. In this context, I also felt that Mr. A was no longer suffering from severe schizophrenia at this point. However, Mr. A says "I'm fine on good days but it's still difficult on bad days. The people in the company are very kind. When I feel bad, they let me take the day off and show flexibility if I am late for work or leave early."

4.1.2 *Details of initial hospitalization*

Mr. A was first hospitalized in his late teens. He says "It started when I heard a conversation between my mother and aunt on a trip to South Korea to visit relatives."

In the conversation, his mother told his aunt that she planned to take out a life insurance policy on Mr. A for 10 million yen. Then, his aunt said to his mother "When you go back to Japan, poison Mr. A." Whether the aunt's comment was true or not, and what her intention was, is not clear, but Mr. A started to distrust others. Even after he returned to live in Japan, he couldn't stop thinking about it, he couldn't eat, and became depressed. According to his psychiatric

DOI: 10.4324/9781003177050-4

diagnosis, hospitalization was recommended, and he was initially admitted. Hospitalization lasted approximately one year.

He was hospitalized for the second time when he was in his early 20s. And this time hospitalization was for one year as well. Mr. A said he did not remember the details of this hospitalization. He was hospitalized a third time while in his late 20s. He became depressed and started to experience auditory hallucinations, and the sounds and music around him seemed to be gossiping and saying bad things about him. He was diagnosed with schizophrenia and hospitalized for approximately one year.

4.1.3 *Family environment*

4.1.3.1 *Presence of the father*

Mr. A's father was born in 1923, in Kyonsannamdo, South Korea. In 1941, at the age of 18, he came to Japan by "conscription." He worked at Miike Coal Mine in Kyushu and was then transferred to Yamaguchi prefecture and the Chubu region. Eventually, he worked in tunnel construction in the Chubu region until the end of the war. He died from liver cancer when he was in his late 60s, when Mr. A was in his mid-teens. Mr. A says all of his father's work sites were oppressive.

> "He sang often. Every time he drank, he would sing. Do you know the song about Miike Coal Mine, 'Tsuki ga detadeta?' There were not only Koreans in 'Takobeya' (harsh labor camps), but also poor Japanese, so I guess he had interactions with Japanese, too. I imagine that they would sing songs like that while laboring together. Yes, from Kyushu, he moved eastward, little by little. (omission) He was brought here to work against his will and was buried alive during tunnel construction. He was trapped in a collapsed mine. He told me the sad story of how difficult it was as he spent three days trapped inside. Maybe it was the same tunnel that he worked on, When the mine collapsed, he suffered a head injury, and he had to care of himself because there was no one to take him to the hospital. Every time he drinks, he talks about his regrets."

Mr. A's parents both remarried when his father was 51, and his mother was 35. At the time, his father already had four daughters, and his mother had a daughter and two sons. Then together, they had Mr. A and his older sister. In other words, Mr. A has four older sisters from a different mother, and an older sister and two older brothers from a different father, and an older sister from the same parents. However, Mr. A actually only lived with his older sister from the same parents.

Mr. A heard from his mother that his father worked for a waste material collection company after the war, and then ran a shipping company. He supposedly made a lot of money while running the shipping company. However, because his father did not receive a school education, he could not read or write. So, the employees were in charge of all the accounting, and one employee stole all the money. The company went bankrupt.

After that, he used the skills he acquired while working during the war and worked for a civil engineering company. As far back as Mr. A remembers, his father was doing this work. Mr. A also remembers that by that time, his father was already an alcoholic and often behaved violently toward his family.

> "I think some people hurt their family due to their mental condition and conduct, and others have been emotionally hurt by the war or other reasons. Accordingly, I wondered about this because my father was like that. He was conscripted and taken to Japan, treated poorly, given insufficient wages. He worked to death, was buried alive, suffered from an accident without paid compensation. He did not have anywhere to release his anger and frustration. Nowhere. Well, that's what I started to think about much later. So he ended up throwing his anger on his family. At home, he somehow tried to cover the pain of his unhealed heart with alcohol, but repeatedly released his frustration by acts of violence toward me, my sister, and my mother. (Omission) Since I was little, how can I say it, inside the house was so tense, it cut through the air. That's why I, myself personally, do not have any freedom. In other words, the reason why I couldn't act voluntarily, and the source of such tense air is from the psychological wounds inflicted by my father and the anger and emotions. We didn't know when he would be in a bad mood."

Mr. A's father also had a gambling addiction. "Almost all the money he made was spent on alcohol and gambling," he said. Of course, his mother had to go to work. "There is no money at home, and we were living practically on my mother's income alone," he said.

4.1.3.2 *Presence of the mother*

Mr. A's mother is now 73 years old and lives alone in Mr. A's home town. She was born on the Korean Peninsula. The Korean War broke out when she was in the 2nd grade of elementary school. Mother's family was poor, living in the countryside, and the people had particularly strong feudalistic thoughts, such as "Women should only work inside the house, only men should study and get a job." His mother "went to school but not regularly," so she does not know how to read Korean nor Japanese.

She often regrets marrying Mr. A's father. She often told Mr. A, "I just married to him following my mother's direction." Mr. A feels "a lack of will and irresponsibility" to his mother.

> "Well, I think if my mother was a person who lived her own life responsibly, she wouldn't say 'Since I was born in South Korea and then came to Japan,

I can't write and understand Japanese of course. So you should help me.' I think that is wrong. It's not my fault she cannot read and write. So much pain, I hated it. Yes, I hated it. She showed me a life insurance contract when I was in the fifth grade of elementary school because she wanted to apply. I had no idea, I was in the fifth grade. Do you think I would be able to understand it? It's complicated. At that time, I wondered what I should do. So, I just said, 'okay, okay.' to get it over with. This isn't what parents are supposed to do to their children, right?"

"What angered me the most was that she sent ambiguous messages to me, because she was still in the role of my mother. Because she couldn't read and write, she told me, 'you are grown up, handle it.' But at the same time, she would tell me 'you will always be a child.' As I received such an ambiguous message, it broke my heart. And she always would tell me, 'Don't be like Aboji (father).' Then when we would fight, she would always say, 'you are just like Aboji' I couldn't handle it, really."

When Mr. A was hospitalized in his early 20s, his mother was also admitted for depression and was hospitalized for approximately one year.

For Mr. A, not only was his father a mental burden, but his mother also subjected him to a negative mental influence.

"Recently this has been termed as 'codependency.' My mother and I were in such a relationship. It was caused by my mother not being able to understand the meaning of her own existence except as a mother, and she could not stop being a mother. In this condition, she could not be independent from me, and many times she would pinch off any new sprouts of my ego. I underwent a form of mental exploitation, and I don't think there was anything in this world with which to judge such mental problems, except by the visible signs of violence."

The above facts indicate that Mr. A was adversely affected by the inseparable condition between mother and son. Therefore, Mr. A was very confused when he heard that his mother had also entered the same hospital. As such he wondered "do I have to meet my mother even if I am hospitalized?" However, their hospital rooms were separated into different wards. He recalls the conditions where he didn't have to meet his mother if he did not actively try was a "good opportunity to consider distancing himself and his relationship with his mother," as compared to when they were living together at home, when maintaining distance was difficult. Currently, he meets his mother once or twice a year when he goes back home.

4.1.4 *Isolation from local society*

There were other Korean families living in the area nearby, but there was no connection between Mr. A's family and other Koreans. There was also an ethnic group association as a local mutual support group for Koreans in the region, but Mr. A's family was poor and could not afford the membership fee, so they could not join the organization. At that time, the sense of discrimination against North/South Koreans was stronger than it is today, and his family was kept at a distance from the surrounding Japanese society and remained isolated. In other words, his family was isolated from both the Zainichi Korean network and the Japanese regional society.

4.1.5 *Meeting with the ethnic group*

Shortly before being hospitalized in his late 20s, Mr. A met a Zainichi Korean ethnic group organization. Here, this organization is described as "N." Mr. A found N by searching the Internet.

> "It was not a Hangul course, what was it at first? I think I participated in something like an exchange festival. Maybe I wanted to connect to a place where the same 'Zainichi' gathered. When I actually went there, I did have a feeling of commonality as a 'Zainichi.' Instead, it was still difficult to find someone to share my feelings with, because there were few people my age with first-generation parents. Maybe second-generation Koreans in their 50s had something in common, but this was not the kind of organization to which those kind of people gathered. My feelings that 'I want to talk about this,' were still not satisfied."

However, Mr. A became more involved with N as the years went by. "I wanted to support N in my own way." However, he says, "I could not talk about part of my experiences in life which I considered important because the people who gathered at N did not have the same kind of problems. If they did, I could make it a topic of conversation. But unfortunately, they didn't. (omission) I didn't feel alienation, but I did feel a bit lonely. Well, what can I say, maybe for me to really be utilized, a person must be able to relate to these kind of problems. Finally... (omission) When I went to N, I was helped to understand why my father was the way he was through various history workshops. However, there wasn't anyone I could talk with about my family issues, my relationship with my mother, and problems like that. In this regard, I read various books, and by reading what was written in these books, I could realize that psychological things cannot be seen. By comparing the cases described in the books and my own experience, I could think that this is the same as me, and that is not. I want to share what caused me to have a mental disorder with more people, and also the relationship between mental disorder and society."

4.1.6 *"The game world"*

> "I love gaming. Gaming is the first place where I could actually feel free in my life. There are rules to the game, but no one complains about what I do as long as l follow the rules. No one laughs when I fail. How can I say?

Anyway, I felt freedom in the game world. I didn't need to worry if someone would complain about what I was doing. I could make mistakes. And if I succeeded, I could feel a sense of accomplishment and fun. I wanted to find a job making video games in the future. So after graduating from junior high school, I started working and went to high school at night. Then I went to a vocational school."

"The game world" was the only time and place where Mr. A felt free. He went to a vocational school for about a year, but then dropped out. After that, he couldn't find employment, got depressed, and started to experience auditory hallucinations. The various sounds around him and the music he heard sounded as if they were gossiping and saying bad things about him. He was diagnosed with schizophrenia and hospitalized for the third time.

In the end, Mr. A said, "I want people to understand how the war affected people living at the time, how it influenced society, families in society, and each individual. And, how to tell that to children. I think it is very important to consider how children will walk in their own life from this time onward."

4.2 Life story of Mr. B

4.2.1 *Family environment*

Mr. B is a man in his late 40s and third-generation Zainichi Korean. A few years ago, he was diagnosed with "bipolar disorder type II." Currently, he has a job, regularly visits a psychiatric clinic, and takes prescribed medicine. His parents are older second-generation Zainichi Koreans. He has an older brother and sister.

Immediately after the war, his father made makkori (Korean distilled spirits) and refined sugar to sell locally and far away towns. Since makkori and refined sugar sold well, Mr. B's family were economically comfortable at that time.

When Mr. B was little, he lived with his paternal grandmother, but she died when he was 8 years old, so he does not remember much about her. The grandmother sold fabric for Chima jeogori (Traditional Korean women's wear) because many Zainichi Korean women still wore ethnic clothes after the war. "My mother said she also received Chima jeogori fabric for her engagement before she got married." With the income from the grandmother, the family was financially comfortable.

Later, they started an "iron company" as suggested by his mother's father, his maternal grandfather. The company would buy scrap metal and sell it to a warehouse dealer. "My mother said it was work Japanese wouldn't do or didn't want to do. Because we were Korean, there was nothing else to do." The business also went comparatively well.

With the resources they accumulated, his father opened a pachinko parlor. Pachinko parlors were still not common at that time. His father's brothers, sisters, and other relatives on his father's side helped and business went well. "That was the best time for our family, wasn't it? That was what I heard. It was before I was born."

Around the time the pachinko parlor business started to take off however, his father became seriously ill and was hospitalized for a year and half. During that time, his relatives took care of the pachinko business, but things didn't go well, and the parlor closed down. "I heard my father deeply regretted that. According to my mother, his personality changed after that. My father invested the money left over after the pachinko parlor closed in stocks. But at that time, Stalin of the Soviet Union died and the stock market crashed, and all the stocks were lost." After a while, his father was discharged from the hospital and he started a printing factory. As far back as Mr. B remembers, his father was doing this work.

"My mother said she hated that job. Because the work was demanding but not profitable. They had to buy expensive equipment, and for less profit. In order to obtain work from the client, they had to buy new equipment to appeal to the client, saying 'We have this equipment, so please give us the work, we can do it.' But the jobs that they received were not so profitable, and as a result, they were left in debt because they bought the equipment."

There were three factories of same business category in the town where his family lived. All of the other owners of the factories were Japanese. "My mother said the big and good jobs were taken by other factories, and the leftover small jobs were given to us. Because we are Korean, it was like, 'If you don't want the job, take it or leave it.'"

Business management was difficult, and the family was always in debt. Of course, the economic condition of the family was hard. "My parents were in a bad relationship; they were always fighting. It was always about business management and debts. So the atmosphere in the house was always negative."

His father did not drink alcohol, but always blamed his mother for "her lack of respect towards him as the family head." And sometimes he behaved violently. "I was never be beaten. My mother said he never behaved violently toward the children. I don't have any memories or remember seeing him behave violently. It sounds like he only behaved violently to my mother. I could tell when I came home after school. Something had happened. The atmosphere was very heavy. My mother was crying. At times like that, I wanted to cry too. One time he poured hot water on her leg. When I came home, my mother was trying to cool her leg. She said one time he beat her, breaking her top front teeth." Inside the house was always negative, Mr. B's family was always afraid of when the father would get angry. "We were relieved when my father left the house. When he was home, the atmosphere was always tense."

Mr. B looks back on his family environment, saying he "could not spend time as a child. Actually, my mother would say 'you should always restrain yourself. Be patient.'"

He remembers being in the fourth grade of elementary school. One day he came home and inside the house was all dark. His older sister was sitting in the living room all alone and looking down quietly. She seemed deep in thought. Then she went to the kitchen and grabbed a knife from under the sink and put it in a drawer. He knew what she was thinking right away. She was planning to stab her father when he came home. Mr. B thought "this is terrible" even though he was still very young. His sister was sitting still and looking down. Since Mr. B was still small, he took out a stool to stand on, removed the knife hidden in the drawer, and returned it under the sink without his sister noticing. She was in the living room, but it was a small room. Mr. B says that his sister probably knew what he was doing behind her back. But she did not stop him.

One time, his mother was abused and ran away. His father noticed and asked Mr. B and his sister, "Where is your mother?" But his sister remained quiet and didn't answer. Once again, Mr. B thought, "this is bad!" and tried to cover things up saying "Didn't she go to visit an aunt living in the nearby town?" He says, "things like that often occurred so I don't have any fond childhood memories." His father died about 20 years ago.

> "My mother says that it is only recently that she and my sister are no longer scared. Even five, six years after my father died, they would still jump every time they heard a noise. When my mother is with my sister, they both become nervous. Because my father behaved violently and raised his voice when he was angry, even after he died, they were afraid every time they heard a strange noise. She said she has finally calmed down. It is the same with me. I still get scared, even now. When I'm startled, it feels a little like I go back to that time. As I listened to what they said, I thought that I was the same."

Mr. B also has the following memories. His father had a younger brother. He was Mr. B's uncle. That uncle always cared for Mr. B's family, providing financial help because he was successful in business. He also took care of Mr. B and his older brother and sister. When he was in elementary school, he would spend his summer vacations at his uncle's house every year. His uncle and aunt knew that his family was not economically comfortable and that Mr. B could not spend his days like a child. They took care of him very much.

> "Summer vacation was when I was set free. I could be free from the dark, heavy, and tense atmosphere of the house. My uncle took good care of me, especially since they still did not have any children, he slept next to me on the bed. But I was scared and couldn't sleep well. It's hard for me to be spoiled."

After staying at his uncle's house until the end of summer vacation, he would return to his own house on the day before the second semester started. The house had a dark and heavy atmosphere as usual.

> "When I went to sleep that night, I cried because I wondered why my house was like this. I was happy this morning and not afraid. Then I came here. I couldn't stop crying. My mother didn't know why I was crying. And she

couldn't ask me gently, 'What's the matter?' 'What happened!' 'Why are you crying?!' She would blame me and hit me on the back. Even I was a child, I remember thinking 'she wouldn't understand.' My mother must have been tired in her everyday life due to her relationship with my father. But, when I learned about father's abuse, I wondered why she would be beaten so severely, such as having her front teeth broken or her leg burned. Why did she put up with it?"

4.2.2 Awareness as a "Zainichi Korean"

Everyone living around Mr. B's house were Japanese. There was almost no interaction with other Zainichi Koreans. His parents hid the fact that "they were Koreans" to other people. As a result, Mr. B also hid his identity as a Korean from his school and friends.

Many Zainichi Koreans lived in the town where Mr. B was born and raised. During the war, there was an ammunitions factory in the town and Koreans were brought over as workers. After the war, many continued to live in the town. Consequently, the neighboring town looked down on Mr. B's town as a "town with many Koreans." The town itself also had strong contempt for Koreans.

Some Korean residential areas in town were called as "Korean communities." The children of Koreans from these areas received blatant discrimination at school. Every time Mr. B saw it, he thought "I should not tell anyone that I am Korean."

Mr. B desperately tried to hide the fact that he was a Korean even more as he grew up. And always "I wanted to become a Japanese. Sometimes, I would even imagine myself as not human, an alien. I look back and laugh at myself, but I was trying to escape from reality. Anyway, I wanted to be a different person. I wanted to escape this environment." he says.

4.2.3 Memories of school education

Mr. B has strong memories of his fifth grade in elementary school.

"I was washing a piece of cloth during cleaning time at school. A girl in the same class came up next to me and started to wash the rags with me. I was excited. Actually, I liked the girl. I was very nervous washing the pieces of cloth together with her but was very happy at the same time. Then she suddenly turned to me and said, 'Are you a Korean?' I got a goose bumps, and it felt as if my hair stood up. I didn't know what to say. Then answered as 'no.' 'I am a mix of Japanese and Korean.' It was a lie. Both of my parents are Zainichi. 'Mix' was a lie, but inside, I knew saying 'Japanese' was a complete lie, but I couldn't say 'Korean' either. So I took the middle course and said 'mixed.' I couldn't say 'I am a Korean.' Even today, I still remember the shock and impact I felt at the time."

Mr. B also remembers the following experience.

"When I was in the sixth grade in elementary school, the teacher liked to have his students write essays, and I wrote an essay for graduation. When the graduation essays were completed, they were distributed to the children. I took them home and showed them to my parents, who had returned from work. I started to leave, when my father said, 'Come here.' My parents were reading the graduation essays, flipping through the pages. Then they said, 'why is only yours like this.' I didn't know. The teacher had re-written all the other students' essays. Only mine was written by hand. I quickly understood what my parents wanted to say. Because my family is Korean, we are treated differently from other children. That was what they wanted to say."

"Of course, now I understand my parent's feelings and why they would say that. My parents were also discriminated against as children. They said people threw stones at them and that they were hurt. That was their generation. That's why they are sensitive about it."

"The class teacher was an old man, but a good teacher. He cared for all the children equally, not only me, without partiality, although he was scary when he got angry. So, when my parents said that, I told them 'that's not the case.' Then my parents said, 'oh, if you say so.' and left it at that."

"But when I went to the school the next day, the teacher called me to the teacher's room after the morning class. There, the teacher's face looked depressed and he said, 'Didn't your parents say something at home yesterday?' I knew right away. 'They had called the school.' But I couldn't say, 'they talked to me,' I answered, 'they didn't say anything.' I don't know why. Since I was a little, I couldn't naturally show my emotions or put them in words. I was torn."

"If I said, 'yes they said something,' the teacher would say 'Yes. actually, your parents called,' but I said 'they didn't say anything,' so he couldn't say much about it. Then the teacher said, 'okay, if you say so.' and that was the end of it."

"During the next class, the teacher told everyone in class. 'There was a mistake in the graduation essay that I passed out, please turn them in again.' The next day, everyone brought their essays and the teacher collected them. A week later, he returned them. I was worried about my essay. I checked it right away. Other children had one correction on their essay, or two at most. But I had three corrections on mine, in the teacher's handwriting. He added three comments, but I felt conflicted. I felt something guilty."

After that, the teacher was transferred to a junior high school in the next town. In junior high school, Mr. B joined the baseball club. And he learned that the teacher had become the coach of the baseball club at the school where he was transferred. Mr. B grew up in a community that formed by combining four towns, including Mr. B's. Once a year, a community baseball game was held.

The main stadium of the community game when Mr. B started junior high school was the school where the teacher was transferred.

On the morning of the day of the game, Mr. B was nervous. Since the graduation essay incident, it would be the first time to see the teacher. He kept wondering how to greet to the teacher and what to talk about if he met the teacher.

That morning, he went to school, walking across the school yard to use the bathroom. Then he saw a man with familiar face walking up to him. It was the teacher. Mr. B kept walking, becoming more and more nervous. His mind was blank. When the teacher approached him, the teacher was smiling. Mr. B smiled back to him. However, they did not exchange words, they just bowed and kept going.

> "The teacher likes physical contact, and often would pat the children on the head and pat them on the shoulder. If the graduation essay incident didn't occur, he would say something like 'how are you doing?' or 'how is junior high school?' patting me on my shoulder or head. I was slightly expecting that. But the graduation essay incident did happen, and because I said 'they did not say anything,' it felt like a bridge that could have been built was suddenly gone between us. An area that was off limits was created. That was why we ended up just bowing and passed by each other. I was very sad."

As Mr. B became a junior high school student, he tried even more desperately to hide the fact that he was Korean. He also worried every day that others would find out.

The town where Mr. B grew up had strong discrimination awareness against Zainichi Koreans. Later Mr. B went to a university in a different region and learned the term "Zainichi Korean." His experiences were called "Zainichi Korean issues," and he learned about education to eliminate these "discrimination issues." However, he never received such education at the school he attended.

In his mathematics class in the April of his first year in junior high school, the first theme was "sets." "Sets" was described as "there is a group called A, and there is a group called B. These are sets." After explaining the general concept of "set," the teacher said, "Ok, can you tell me some kinds of sets we have, one by one?" The students were called on to answer, and it was the student sitting right behind Mr. B's turn. The student said, "Nationalities!"

In April, students from elementary school are just coming to junior high school. The word "nationality" was not too familiar to those children. Students in class were perplexed and were asking each other, "what's that?" However, Mr. B fully understood "nationality."

From his attitude toward Mr. B, it seems that the student knew Mr. B was Korean. Mr. B thinks the student said "nationality!" to tell him, "I know who you are."

At the time, Mr. B's hair stood up and he got goose bumps. He feared the other student was asking, "Are you Korean?" However, all he could do was look natural so others wouldn't notice. Mr. B says, "Students who know I am Korean always know my 'weakness.' I was always worried that they would tell others. So, I always tried to gain their favor. I had a very subservient attitude."

I also didn't expect the mathematic teacher's reaction. When the student said "Nationality!", the teacher was embarrassed and panicked saying, "Don't say that!" The other students looked confused.

> "They had no idea of the meaning of 'nationality' nor why the teacher got upset and said 'don't say that!' Later, I thought this was very symbolic. In other words, in that town, the topic of nationality, which meant Korean, was something which should be mentioned. I think the attitude of the teacher expressed this quite well."

Mr. B also remembers the following. Although not required in school education today, but at the time, Mr. B's school required students to submit a document called a "personal statement." In that document, matters of personal privacy, such as domicile of origin, family composition and occupation of parents, were listed on the cover page. This "personal statement" was returned to the student at each semester every year, and the student was required to update the information and resubmit it. This was very painful for Mr. B. The problem was how the document was collected.

> "When collecting the 'personal statement,' students in each column were told to 'pass it from the back, to the person in front' just like collecting a test paper. Everyone would place his own paper on top of the paper from the student behind him. That meant the student in front of me would see the cover page of my personal statement. On my cover page, "Korea" is written in the "domicile of origin" column. The fact that I was Korean could be exposed."

So others would not find out Mr. B was Korean, every semester, as the classroom would get noisy and the student sitting in front of him turned around to get Mr. B's statement, Mr. B would get that student's personal statement first and put it on top of his statement, and then take the statements to the student sitting two rows ahead. How to do this "unusual action" naturally was his critical mission each semester. Every time he did that, he worried if others would see his cover page. As mentioned earlier, the town where Mr. B grew up, and the school he attended, had strong discrimination awareness toward Zainichi Koreans. The psychology of Korean children was not understood at all, and school education was developed without such consideration. Mr. B says "I've heard that things still haven't changed." For Mr. B, the words and characters for "Korea" and "Korean" were loathed.

> "In junior high and high school history textbooks, the 'Joseon Dynasty' is mentioned. It is also listed on the Table of Contents. When I would see

that, I hated it and was even afraid of it. When I wrote a diary, etc. I wanted to write about my anxieties about being Korean. But I cannot even write the word 'Korean.' I am afraid of those characters. So, I would use a black marker and cross out the word 'Korea' in the textbook. Sometimes if there were too many, I would glue the pages together."

Mr. B went to a high school in the town next to the one where he was born and raised. His life worrying about whether others would learn that he was a Korean still didn't change. Outwardly, he smiled and appeared calm, always serious and with high standards. He pretended to live like a Japanese so people wouldn't say "because he's Korean," when they found out. "So honesty, I didn't know who I was anymore. I don't know even now." he says.

As a result, when Mr. B looks at his high school graduation album, he feels strange. It's strange to see himself in the class photo. In addition, he is surprised that he doesn't remember his high school days, he has no memories of them.

Friends who didn't know that Mr. B was Korean, would make discriminating remarks about the many Koreans in their town and about Koreans themselves. Mr. B could only laugh and go along. However, among the few memories he does have, one strongly remains. It is about a book report in his second year in high school.

"My summer vacation homework was a book report. I read 'Hakai' (meaning of "break the commandments) of Toson Shimazaki. It's a story about community issues. The main character, Ushimatsu Segawa, comes from a discriminated community. He is a teacher and hides where he came from. After reading 'Hakai,' what remains in my heart the most down to this day is that it was painful for Ushimatsu Segawa to hide this fact from others. He is afraid that others will find out one day. And he tries to get rid of his fear and sadness by drinking alcohol with someone, such as a coworker. He drinks too much and gets drunk. He wants to cry so much; he can't help it. But instead of crying, he looks up to the ceiling and laughs out loud. He laughs, instead of crying. When a person is deep in despair, he can't cry. Tears don't fall. He can only laugh. When I read that part, I couldn't stop crying. I was definitely Ushimatsu. I couldn't stop crying."

The book report was supposed to 400 words, 5 pages or less. However, Mr. B wrote 15 pages. "Hakai" left that strong of an impression.

At the time, Mr. B was class representative. One of his roles was to collect the book reports from the students and take them to the teacher in charge of the "Japanese" class. He took the book reports to the teacher's room and gave them to the teacher in charge. The book reports were arranged in order of the students' numbers in the class. The teacher in charge said "thank you," and immediately started reading the book reports. Mr. B's student number just happened to be near the top. After the teacher looked at some of the students' book reports, he set them aside, but when he came to Mr. B's report, he started to read it. Since the teacher was not his homeroom teacher, he didn't know that the book report was written by the student who had just delivered it. When Mr. B saw that the teacher had started to read his own book report, he "slipped away and left."

The next time class was held by the teacher, the class started as usual. Mr. B was called on to answer a question and stood up. Then the teacher said, "Are you the one who wrote about 'Hakai?'" Mr. B answered, "Yes." The teacher said in front of the whole the class, "There will be a book report contest for the prefecture, I would like to submit yours, to represent this school. You did a great job." This caused a stir among the students. Mr. B felt "a mix of happiness and shame."

Why did the teacher do that? Mr. B says,

> "Maybe the teacher asked the homeroom teacher about me. Then found out that I am a Korean. A Korean student reads about community issues in 'Hakai' and writes a book report. And writes something very emotional. Of course, while pretending to be Japanese. I think the teacher was trying to encourage me. Like 'Things happen, but do your best.' I guess that's what it means. This is one of the few happy memories I have of high school."

He has a few happy memories like that, "but my younger days were dark."

In high school, his life was a little rough. He stopped going to school a couple of times. Many nights, he would ride a male relative's motorcycle without his permission around town and ended up being chased by a police car. One cold day, he rode into a shopping arcade and hid behind a table in front of a store for about an hour until the police car left.

> "I didn't use thinner, but almost did. My parents were very confused. Up to then, I was a 'serious boy.' 'What happened?' As I look back, I didn't have any hope of the future."

Mr. B has an older brother and sister. When Mr. B was an elementary school student, his brother graduated from the university. As an outstanding student, his older brother was almost hired by a major trading company. A university alumnus working at the company guaranteed, "you will definitely be hired." His brother went to the interview but wasn't hired. His brother and family were sure he would be hired, so they were very disappointed with the results. Later, the alumni came to his house to explain what happened. Nationality was the issue. "There is nothing wrong with you, but your nationality was the problem."

When this is the conversation, the question from Japanese society always comes up. "Why didn't you obtain Japanese nationality?" However, it's not that simple. Obtaining Japanese nationality, also called naturalization, is a high hurdle. It is also an emotional issue for Zainichi Koreans. At the time, it was harder than it is now. "Why didn't you obtain Japanese nationality?" If someone asks such a question, it means he doesn't understand the circumstances and history of

Zainichi Koreans. Mr. B's older brother B was disappointed and left for a while. No one knows where he went.

Mr. B's older sister was in a romantic relationship with a Japanese man, and both of them wanted to get married. But his family opposed, and they gave up. She and her mother cried for days.

Mr. B saw such unhappiness in his family all through his childhood. It was not "the person's fault" or "lack of effort," but just the fact that they were Korean, they lost out on opportunities to get a job or get married. Mr. B has seen it since he was little. Mr. B says, "When I saw it, I thought, I will face the same things when I grow up. And was afraid to become an adult."

All of his classmates in high school painted their own future vision, such as "I want to go to that university," "after I graduating from the university, I want to get this kind of job." However, Mr. B could not paint such a vision.

> "I started to think, even if I study hard and get good grades, people will still say no, 'because I am Korean,' Trying is meaningless, it's better not to try. So I became desperate."

4.2.4 *Awareness of illness*

Mr. B said he was aware that he had a disorder since he was young. His oldest memory is when he was a high school student, he already felt intense waves of emotion. He could act cheerfully when in high spirits, but after that, "I would suddenly realize in my head that this is not the real me, then get so depressed that I couldn't get up." Most people thought he was a "calm person," but once he got angry, he would become so furious that people would say "I can't believe (he) is the same person." Mr. B suffered from his own personality since he was young. He wondered, "Why can others live in such a stable condition, without any waves?"

Five years ago, Mr. B experienced severe depression as never before. "The direct cause was a personal relationship related to work. I took a break for a while because I couldn't get up."

Later, he returned to the work, but could tell that he would get angry even over small matters. "Inside my head, my logic would tell me I shouldn't say anything, but I couldn't control myself and would say it anyways. I thought I couldn't control myself. If this continues, it's not good."

Then he visited a psychiatric clinic. He was first diagnosed with "minor depression" and given a medicine prescription. However, he didn't feel like he was getting better.

So he started to read books on mental disorders and found the word "bipolar disorder." As he looked at the listed symptoms, he thought "Doesn't this describe me?" He told that to the attending physician, but the doctor said, "lining up these disorders is difficult."

Mr. B was introduced to a clinic specializing in the study of bipolar disorders. He visited the clinic and received a test that identifies diseases by analyzing the blood flow in the brain. As a result, he was diagnosed with "a mood disorder" and "bipolar disorder Type II." When he received the diagnosis, he says "I found myself relieved. This isn't my personality, but an illness." Since then, he regularly visits the clinic and receives his medicine prescription.

4.2.5 *Suicide attempt*

Mr. B suffered "intense waves of emotion" since he was young. He could work smoothly when his condition was good, but if his condition worsened, he would become depressed. And, when he was in a poor condition, he would easily become angry, and could not control his anger. One moment he would think he could do something "smoothly," but the next day his condition would usually get worse. This kept repeating.

Mr. B continued to hide the fact that he is a Korean, even after he left his hometown to go to the university. He did not tell his friends while attending the university. When he looked for part-time work, and sought employment, he was often turned down because "Korea" was written on his resume. When he was looking for a place to rent, he often encountered "No Koreans." When he told a woman whom he started dating that "he was Korean," she stopped seeing him saying "my parents are sensitive about it." Mr. B says, "Things are no different than when my parents were young. Conditions are still bad, and I can't do anything about. That's just the way it is."

Mr. B attempted suicide two times when he was in early 20s. Both times he felt hopeless due to receiving such discriminatory treatment. And both times, he caused an accident by not stopping his car behind the line at an intersection but stepping on the accelerator. His car lunged forward and was hit by a car from the side. One time, the whole car was thrown into the air and flipped over. Miraculously, he only suffered minor injuries. "At that time, I thought I could die. I feel so sorry for the person in the other car. It was a disaster. I'm lucky to be alive today."

> "I have dated but have repeatedly ruined the relationship because of my hot temper. A person who is always calm, all of a sudden becomes angry one day. The other person must not know what to do. One person said that she "was afraid because she didn't know when she might push the wrong button and anger me." That is why, I think living with someone and getting married is difficult. I don't have any children, and I think it's better that I don't. But I do like children. If I have children, I would be like my father. I think my children would be terrified of me. So, I am glad that I don't have any children."

Mr. B says that he has dreams about his father even now. "It's always a 'scary dream.' The other day, I dreamt he pushed me off a stone wall of a castle."

Since he started taking medicine, he feels the intense waves of emotion are under control for the first time. However, he still has good and bad days. He spends much of his time alone, because he would bother others.

4.3 Life story of Mr. C

Mr. C is a man in his early 50s. He is "half Japanese, half Korean" with a first-generation Zainichi Korean father and Japanese mother. His sister is 12 years older than him. His first diagnosis was "depression," "severe stress disorder with mood disorder," and "PTSD." Currently, he holds a health handbook designating him as disabled.

Recently, rather than using terms such as "half" or "mixed blood," which often are used with a negative connotation when referring to persons born from an international marriage, the term "double," which has a positive meaning, has begun to be heard more often. However, such persons themselves have expressed the opinion that terms like "half" or "person of mixed blood" should be strategically and positively used in order to describe their suppressed and surrounding circumstances.

In line with this movement, the term "half" is used here because Mr. C, the survey subject, refers to himself as such.

In addition, Mr. C, who is half Japanese, half Korean, identifies his physical gender and sexual identity as transgender. The target of romantic intentions are women, but since his gender identity is "female," he considers himself as a homosexual. Mr. C lives with such a complex identity. All last names described below are pseudonyms.

4.3.1 *Family environment*

Mr. C's father was born in South Korea in 1917 and is a first-generation Zainichi Korean who came to Japan in 1935. He passed away in 1969, when Mr. C was 7 years old. He died suddenly when his peritonitis worsened. He collapsed and was taken to the hospital but died three days later. Mr. C's mother is Japanese, born in 1925, and died in 1990 at the age of 65.

His parents did not file marriage papers but had "a common-law marriage" as coined these days. The reason for this was that they wanted their children to have Japanese citizenship since they lived in Japan. Since Mr. C was born under the former Citizenship Law (based on the citizenship of one's father, only if the father was Japanese could his children obtain Japanese citizenship), he would automatically receive foreign citizenship because his father was not a Japanese. To avoid that, they decided to have a common-law marriage. His mother submitted the birth notification and registered him under her family registry, without submitting a marriage notification. In the registry of a child of unmarried mother, the column of father is left blank, and the child is not described as "first son/daughter" etc., but simply as "male/female" (after 2004, this can be changed by application to change the description to "first son/daughter," etc. Mr. C changed his status to first son, by his own will.)

Consequently, Mr. C's nationality since birth was listed as "Japanese" according to his mother's nationality. Moreover, his father's last name was "Kim" and his mother's was "Tanaka." But since common law marriages were looked down upon, the whole family lived under his father's Japanese last name, "Suzuki," to avoid discrimination. Mr. C's father owned a factory making machinery screws. However, he died "before determining whether the business was established or not."

> "He was a serious person. He played a little when he was young, but later he was serious. Maybe because we were born. It sounds like he became serious since then. When he was alive, we weren't 'rich,' but we could live comfortably. We had a dog, a Japanese Spitz, which was rare at the time. There weren't many Spitz back then. I guess we had a good life. My mother was a housewife but started to work at home after my father died. She raised us by herself. She often talked about our father."

Mr. C lost his father when he was 7, and his maternal grandfather who was living in the same house died soon after. Losing his father and grandfather greatly affected Mr. C's state of mind, and this triggered him to become "closed-off."

4.3.2 Realization of being "half Japanese, half Korean" and awareness of sexual discomfort

Mr. C attended elementary school under his father's Japanese name, "Suzuki." However, his name on his health insurance card was "Tanaka," his registered family name. At the time, Mr. C was confused, "not knowing which name is my real name." In 1974, when he entered junior high school, he told his mother that he would use his name "Tanaka" at school, because he didn't like "the confusion about which is his real name."

"Names" are a complicated issue for a Zainichi Korean. Until recently, a Zainichi Korean could change his Japanese name (common name). Many Zainichi Koreans changed their common name due to various situations in their lives. Children do not understand these situations faced by adults. The issue of one's name confuses children, such as why the name they usually use and the name on their health insurance card differ. When they go to school, friends are suspicious and say, "why did you change your name?" "Why did you change your Kanji (Chinese characters)?" However, children do not understand the reasons. For many children who lived their lives unaware that they are "Zainichi," it is even more difficult to explain.

At the age of 16, when Mr. C asked his mother as "when anxiety about his name reached the limit," he was told for the first time that his father was Korean. Even though his father was a first-generation Zainichi, his Japanese was very fluent. As a result, Mr. C did not know that his father was "not Japanese." When his mother told him, Mr. C had no idea where "South Korea" was and was caught totally unaware.

When he heard that, Mr. C's natural reaction was to be "happy as a child of an international marriage." When he told one of his close friends, the friend asked, "why you didn't get naturalized?" Another friend said, "why did you tell me?" He did not care.

After Mr. C found out his father was Korean, and that he himself was half Japanese, half Korean, he started reading books related to North and South Korea in the library. However, at the time in 1978, even though there were some books about Zainichi North and South Koreans, there was nothing describing "halfs" like Mr. C.

He finally found a sentence in one book – "the topic of children with mixed blood has been taboo in Zainichi society." At that time, Mr. C "became frightened and felt intense ostracism." And, he began to doubt, "who am I?" and was distressed for many days. He describes his mental state as "I liked both Japan and Korea but hated them at the same time."

On the other hand, his memory of gender dysphoria began when he was 4 years old. He says, "The trigger was I found myself feeling comfortable when I playing with girls. I was strongly interested in playing house and wanted to wear a skirt. And it was very difficult to control my desire to act like a girl. I also wanted to wear red clothes but couldn't say it. There was common sentiment that red is for girls, blue for boys."

4.3.3 *Awareness of discrimination against "Zainichi Koreans"*

When Mr. C was 18 years old, he attended a vocational design school, because he liked to draw pictures. However, he quit after a year. After that, he started to become aware of "discrimination against Zainichi North/South Koreans," and became hikikomori (acute social withdrawal).

His mother died when he was 28 years old. At his mother's funeral, he heard his relatives talking to each other saying that "she shouldn't have married such a person," something that he never heard before. He was shocked. "I was surprised to know that Japanese look down on Japanese who are married to Koreans. In other words, Japanese discriminate against Japanese."

> "My relatives were appalling. Their attitude suddenly changed, right after my mother died. They said that on the day of the funeral. They didn't say such terrible things while my mother was alive, but as soon as she died... I was surprised. Marrying a Korean must be uncomfortable for them. Only my sister and her husband interact with our family relatives. They were the only people who met together. Because my mother married a Korean, I think our family was outside the relatives' circle. We were isolated from our relatives. So I never played or had interactions with my cousins."

Mr. C asked his sister and relatives about making a grave for his parents, but they immediately rejected it saying, "it's not necessary." Mr. C thought the reason behind it was the fact that his father was Korean. He felt "there's discrimination even when making a grave."

His sister didn't tell her husband's father and his family that her father was Korean. Her husband was also strongly opposed to making a grave saying, "from the public viewpoint, openly exposing this is not good." However,

Mr. C did not want to give up on his parents' grave and decided to build it himself.

4.3.4 *Complicated identity*

However, Mr. C attempted suicide when he was 32. "I walked around town each night and climbed up to the top of a building with an iron tower to jump off and die but couldn't kill myself." The day before he decided to commit suicide, he wrote a suicide note and posted it at the branch of "an ethnic organization" near his house, the Zainihon-Daikanminkoku-Mindan (An organization made up of Koreans in Japan who support South Korea). He then climbed up the iron tower to jump but couldn't, so he went to the ethnic organization to apologize. When Mr. C went to apologize, the branch chief responded. The branch chief was Zainichi Korean, and the first whom Mr. C met after his father.

> "I went there the day after I couldn't commit suicide. I think the branch chief came out. He told me not to die. He said his son had died in a construction accident. He told me not to die because he also had a similar experience. But I haven't seen him since then."

Why would Mr. C leave a suicide note in "the ethnic organization's" office?

> "I wanted them to know that there people like me. I wanted to leave something behind. Because I felt that only 'Zainichi' see other 'Zainichi'. 'Halfs' never appear in books written by 'Zainichi', so I am saddened that our existence is ignored. I felt like halfs existed below 'Zainichi' society, something like 'an appendage.' I feel like halfs appear only when convenient, such as bringing out a half to promote the end of discrimination, something like 'let's aim for a society of coexistence.' I think Zainichi society is narrow-minded. I feel uncomfortable because I think 'Zainichi' talk about halfs within the range of 'Zainichi society.' A person like me doesn't have a place in Japan, but there isn't a place for me in Zainichi society either. That's why I thought about leaving 'my fingernail marks' at the nearby ethnic organization although I had never contacted it. At least before I die. In the letter I also wrote, 'sorry I couldn't build his grave,' to my father's relatives in South Korea, whom I had never met. I thought the ethnic organization could send it."

When Mr. C was young, the term "sexual identity disorder" did not exist. Mr. C also suffered and was troubled by his own sexuality. As he worried about being "half Japanese, half Korean" and his sexuality, he was mentally cornered and couldn't consult with anyone. He started to think "I must be crazy." He attempted suicide again in his early 30s.

When he was 33, he worked at pachinko parlor. He wanted to have "Zainichi" friends, but all his coworkers were Japanese. A coworker said, "He's Korean" and the chief said, "we don't need any foreigners." He also had the experience that the owner of the Japanese pub that he regularly visited was obviously upset when he talked about "ethnicity."

To forget such anxieties regarding his ethnic origin, Mr. C became obsessed and addicted to pachinko, regularly went to "sex establishments," and became burdened with debt. His pachinko addiction continued for 4–5 years. Depression developed and he was treated by a psychiatrist. He was diagnosed with "depression," "severe stress disorder with mood disorder," and "PTSD." Mr. C told the attending physician about his background and sexuality. Later, the appearance of strong anxiety symptoms of "not knowing who he is" was considered to be caused by the mourning of the death of a parent from a sensitive childhood age of seven, followed by learning that he was "half Japanese half Korean," along with "the complicated conditions" of feeling discomfort with one's own gender at an early age.

> "This is my experience as a child. Fear of death was burned into my mind. I feel that is the source of my illness. I am afraid of death, but my mind is drawn to suicide. I myself don't understand. In the movie 'Sonatine' directed by Takeshi Kitano, the main character with suicidal ideas has the line, 'if you are so afraid of dying, you want to die even more.' I think that's it."

Even with such difficult experiences, Mr. C could still save his money, accumulating 1 million yen for his parents' grave by the time he was 37. And he established a grave in a famous temple in Kansai. He had both of his parents' names on the grave. For his father's name, both his Japanese name and his Korean name were written and included "Hongan" with the Korean name. "Hongan (hometown)" is used to describe the birthplace of founder of a family or clan, it is very significant in the family system in South Korea, even today.

Mr. C was adamant on building his parents' grave because he wanted to do it "for them." His mother kept his father's remains at home.

> "I think they were a good couple. I wanted a grave just for them. I won't be put in there. I'm a good-for-nothing son, I don't think I'm qualified to be there. So, as a couple's grave, it would be a permanent memorial at the temple. The temple said they will keep them even after I die, so I decided to place them there. I haven't seen them recently, though. I go once every two or three years. (omission) When I talked to the gravestone mason, he said, 'this cemetery has many graves of local North/South Koreans. There are some people like you, who place the real names on the grave so that the nationality is clearly visible, and then there are some people who don't have any traces of the country they came from, so that the grave looks exactly like a Japanese grave. There is a stark division. One or the other.'"

When Mr. C built his parents' grave, his sister told certain members of her in-laws that her father was a Korean for the first time. His sister lives "like a perfect Japanese." But Mr. C "wants to live as a half." Still, he attempted suicide again after that.

> "My goal in life was to build my parents' grave. But once that was accomplished, I lost the will to live. It's called the 'burn out syndrome.'"

He was once again "disappointed because I don't know who I am," but stopped himself just before jumping off the building. He did this repeatedly. He then became homeless and was sleeping in a riverbed.

When he was 38, he started to do day work at a construction site. And at 41, he became "a part-time leader" at the site and found a girlfriend.

He was hesitant to tell her that he was half Japanese half Korean, but when he told her, she was 16 years younger and showed "understanding" without discrimination. At 44 years old, Mr. C became engaged with the woman. After the engagement, he told her parents that he is half Japanese half Korean and they understood, but her younger brother clearly showed an unpleasant look.

However, Mr. C still did not tell her that he had bouts of depression. When he told her this, she couldn't accept it, and the engagement was canceled.

> "She really wanted to have children. Maybe after repeatedly hearing about the psychiatric clinic and my depression, she became worried about it being hereditary."

When he was 45, his symptoms of depression worsened, and he received psychiatric treatment.

4.3.5 *Current conditions*

Mr. C is certified as a person with a mental disorder, and regularly visits a daycare center affiliated with the hospital for people with mental disorders and alcohol dependency. Mr. C lives with multiple marginality, such as half Japanese half Korean, transgender, and mental disorder. He "thinks there is no cure" for his own illness. But he started to think that he "originally lived with mental disease," and he could feel a little better when he changed his way of thinking.

The attending physician at the hospital and the physician of the daycare hospital are different. Mr. C found that psychiatrists view transgenders differently. The attending physician is a woman, she listens and understands his talk, and writes down details on his chart. However, the male physician at the daycare told him "don't talk to others at the daycare about it, and I'm not going to write it down on the chart either." After that, Mr. C hasn't talked about his sexuality.

Mr. C started to use the Internet around 2003. The famously "huge bulletin board" was full of discriminatory words. Therefore, he tried not to see entries of discrimination against Zainichi Koreans. When he reads a discriminatory entry, he starts to hyperventilate, becomes physically weak, and his depression symptoms worsen. And, he has nightmares at night. The physicians even told him not to view such entries. In recent years, when he sees demonstrations by hate groups on the Internet, he experiences symptoms such as he cannot move his body.

To encourage himself, he "manages a blog that clearly states a person's real name, origin, and address." He thinks "maybe because the blog is like that, only serious comments without discrimination are made. Most are from women and all are Japanese. I wonder if discrimination of foreigners is predominately by men." He feels "Japan is a country where men control the political culture and environment, superiority of men over women is still strong, and this male dominated society is basically exclusive. In contrast, women maybe easy-going and have less discrimination, and many are gentle." "Easy-going without discrimination, that's my mother."

> "I read the book, 'Organization to restore ethnic names' in the late 1980s. The words, 'standing in Japanese society and showing ourselves just as we are is important,' left a strong impression on my heart. That's why I have a blog in my real name. When I see someone anonymously demanding the outlawing of the common name of a 'Zainichi', I naturally feel it's a contradiction. Actually, I almost want to laugh. Revealing one's real name is very risky and scary. If I try to change jobs and have an interview, the person from the human resources department will search for my name and find my blog, that's also frightening. But I think of myself having an honest blog with my real name is motivated by something that is not wrong and want to live that way. I'm sure I'll live a hard life."

"I have conflicting emotions. I love Japan and Korea, but I also hate Japan and Korea." Mr. C heard that persons who are half Japanese half Korean in South Korea also suffer discrimination. As a result, he has "anti-Korea" feelings within himself.

He wants to publicize his own origins as "half Japanese half Korean" at every opportunity, not just on the Internet, but also in real society. He actually announced such, but also experienced "anxiety at the same time."

Mr. C is proud that he is "half," but is unable to join "Zainichi society." "I always feel a 'wall' between myself and 'Zainichi society.' 'Zainichi' talk about 'halfs' with sensitivity and logic while keeping themselves in the center. I feel strong discomfort and rejection." He is still unclear about his own social position, even when he goes for a walk, he remembers discriminatory words and actions, becomes confused, feels pain, and then squats down.

A big change, a turning point, came in 2015. He always wanted to work for other people, so he obtained a certificate, "Beginner's training seminar for long-term care work," despite having mental disorders. And, at the same time, he regularly went to a Catholic Christian baptism course. He became a Christian the following year. Since Christianity teaches "suicide is prohibited," he no longer dwells on suicide. His mental state is one of "I want to live," and "I am not good at connecting with people, but I love them."

"Through the Internet environment I obtained since 2003, I have been able to connect with real people, and this has greatly changed me. Through the Internet, several people have become my real friends. I started to participate in social exchanges held by a LGBT organization over the Internet, and after exchanges with people with physical disabilities whom I met over the Internet, I thought about obtaining a nursing care license. Originally, I was not good at human relationships. So, I always wanted to overcome this by utilizing the Internet."

When he was 4 years old, a picture of the Virgin Mary was hanging in a room. It left a strong impression on his mind. Mr. C took a few baptism courses in the year his mother died but stopped going because he thought "it is not appropriate for such a disobedient child as me." 25 years later, he searched for peace in his heart, and decided to get baptized without telling the church that he is transgender. He got baptized a year later. Later, he was relieved to know there was a Christian group who considered LGBT issues.

"Different from young halfs, double-mix, and quarters today, I have some very old discrimination experiences. There is a generation gap, and I feel like I am a pretty old-fashioned half, a stubborn type, a 'dark half.' I hate myself. It's ok to bring up the painful past, but this is too much. I find myself stuck in the past that I hate. I wish I were the last 'half' who writhes in agony. Some people are still discriminated against and become paranoid. Actually, I have that tendency, so I am careful to avoid it and try to find something fun because I want to live a cheerful life. Isolation as a minority is scary. It is better to use the Internet and/or SNS if you can, even with their many problems. These days, you can find friends over the Internet, and can find common ground with various types of people. There must be something better. (omission) I experienced mental disorders since I was a child and is currently 54 years old. Even if I am discriminated against by others, I am proud of being 'half Japanese, half Korean.' Still, I sometimes introduce myself as 'a child of immigrants,' instead of half Japanese, half Korean. These days, I think this word fits me better. Actually, the issue in terms of address, such as 'half, double, and mix,' should be decided by each individual personally, and not by others. So I think they are all correct, even though they differ by individual. But if you really think about it, none of the terms 'half, double, and mix' were actually coined by the persons themselves. These words were decided by other people according to how they viewed us. (omission) Japan has not been at war for decades and is considered to be a peaceful country. But why is it still so difficult to live? For Japanese people as well as for us?"

Even now, Mr. C has difficulty talking to others one to one. At the daycare center, 80% of his conversations are with women. He is terrified to talk to men and has a strong tendency to avoid talking to them. He has a deep-seated fear of men and thinks this is due to men more frequently making discriminatory remarks. He thinks of himself as "a minority among a minority," a person with mental disorders, half Japanese, half Korean, and transgender.

4.4 Life story of Mr. D

Mr. D was born in the 1950s and is a second generation of Zainichi Korean. At the time of the interview, he was in his 60s. After graduating from a university, he worked full time at a Zainichi Korean ethnic organization. Due to various experiences at work, he developed symptoms of mental disorder in his 20s. In some ways, his experience and onset process are representative of the experiences of second-generation Zainichi Koreans who grew up in the 1960s and 70s and were influenced by the political conditions between three nations – Japan, South Korea, and North Korea.

Mr. D also repeatedly attempted suicide. Currently, he regularly visits a medical clinic, and takes medicine to sleep, as needed. He is also a member of an NPO (Nonprofit Organization) that supports persons with mental disorders and spends his local life with the mutual support of friends.

4.4.1 *Family environment*

The interview was carried out at Mr. D's home. His residence is 12 tsubo (39.6 m) wide and is located at the corner of a long house. Mr. D was born in a nearby house, but soon after his birth, his family moved to his current residence.

The area where he lives is one where many Koreans lived after the war. That reputation still remains today, but as the generation passes, many "Zainichi" have left the area and the current "Zainichi" population has decreased.

There are his parents, six brothers and sisters, and himself in his family.

His father was born in the 1910s on Jeju Island. His mother was also born on Jeju Island in the same year. His parents got married on Jeju Island. The marriage was arranged by their parents. His father came to Japan when he was around 20 years old. He was the youngest son in his family. Life in his hometown was nearly self-sufficient. They lived by eating fish they caught themselves, as well as millet, oats, etc. Since Mr. D's father had other brothers, he came to Japan to earn money for his parents.

> "My father attended school but did not receive any higher education. He had good penmanship. He was also good at calligraphy. Many people from Jeju island live in Osaka because it is a direct ship route. When moving to a foreign country, one will often live where they know someone, or around those from the same village. After settling into his life to a certain extent, my mother came to Japan."

Mr. D's father came to Japan and worked for a textile company. At the time, Japan was experiencing economic prosperity, and his salary was high. His father sent money he had earned to his parents in his hometown. "I think he just wanted do a lot for his parents. Maybe that was what he was thinking." He did not have a muscular build, so manual labor was difficult for him. Mr. D does not remember well, but after working at the factory for a few years, his father became independent.

> "My father was working for textile business, maybe plastics as well. Are you familiar with Bakelite? It's a plastic. Japan seemed to have greatly profited from the textile business at that time. After the war, we moved five minutes away to this residence. Only this room had a tiled roof, and here was like a garden. Our family all lived here together, nine people. Really. We lived here."

Mr. D's father was a gentle and serious worker. Mr. D has no recollection of his father hitting him. His father never drank alcohol, he was gentle and had a sense of humor, as was his mother. "They had gentle personalities. They were never mean to me." His family got along well. His oldest brother was an outstanding person. He knew a lot about machines. Because the family could not live solely on the family business, the oldest son worked as a homeschool teacher. The second son was 8 years older than Mr. D, and was the only one to graduate junior high school and started to work at a factory.

At the time, few Zainichi Koreans went to high school. Many went to work after finishing junior high school. Since the family was poor, the second brother could not go on the school trip to Tokyo. In addition, two other "Zainichi" students who lived in the neighborhood also could not go. These students went to school instead.

All of Mr. D's brothers and sisters were aware that their parents were burdened with debt from the business and thought they would have to work together to pay back the debts after graduating from school. In addition, "we were saying to each other that after we pay off the debts, let's build a two-story house for us all to live in."

However, managing a private business was difficult and the family was poor. "There were always debts, we had to pay back the money." His parents received money from Tanomoshikou (a private mutual aid organization for financial interchange) and bought machines for their privately owned factory. Tanomoshikou is a long established private financial union in Japan that is managed by an association organization. Members contribute regular installments and then one of the members receives a specified amount of money as determined by bidding or lottery each time. Once all the members have been paid, the association is dissolved. The collected money is used to buy livestock, household goods, etc. There are various methods, one for example is when a person who needs the money becomes the "parent" and is called Tanomoshi. Then, the association members would each pay a certain amount of money. Next, those members who need money would bid on how much interest they could pay, such as "I will pay this much interest, please give the money to me." The person who bids the highest interest rate will receive the pooled money, and then pay the money back to each association member. Zainichi Koreans also used this Tanomoshikou to pay for living expenses and obtain working capital for business.

His father was a serious worker, but Mr. D says he thinks his father didn't want to deal with money payments and didn't have business savvy. As a result, his mother always went to pay the Tanomoshikou with money she had earned. His mother did all the work. After one job finished, she worried if the next job was coming or not. Since Koreans could not borrow money from the bank, they had no choice but to obtain money from cooperative associations such as Tanomoshikou.

> "Tanomoshikou is illegal today. People pay several 10,000 yen each month. 10 to 20 people are gathered and each contributes a certain amount, then each month, someone would receive it. During that time, we didn't have room to pay the money, so we would always have to accept any work. So even if the interest rate was high, we had to quickly raise our hand and take the job. My mother did everything. My father just worked morning to night, that was all he did. We would have some Tanomoshikou payments each month. Without exception. We were always living with heavy hearts and anxiety, and worried if the next job would come and were pressed for the next payment."

At first, his father, brothers, and mother worked using hand-operated machines. The machines were gradually updated to semi-automatic machines, and then fully automated in the 1970s, when Mr. D was a university student. While Mr. D was preparing to re-take the university entrance examination, he also helped with the work.

In the early 1970s, the initial salary of a university graduate was 30,000–40,000 yen. But during that time, the family could earn up to hundreds of thousands of yen from a job. On the other hand, work conditions were extremely difficult, and the machines were operated from 8 am until 11 pm, without a day off. Still, depending on the job, new machines were needed. At first, the machines cost about 500,000 yen per unit. However, as performance increased, the cost of the machines also climbed into the millions of yen. The family needed new machines, but they didn't have the money to buy them, so purchases were made using Tanomoshikou. The family consecutively purchased 4–5 units of expensive machinery. Of course, the amount of repayment for Tanomoshikou also increased, and most of the money they earned went to those payments. "Although we worked from morning to evening, it seemed like we were working to pay the interest on the loans, working to pay back other people, working so others could make a profit. I saw this since I was a child, and the level of poverty was severe. We were really poor. But I thought being poor was normal."

According to "History Textbook-Zainichi Korean History" (2013), discrimination against Zainichi Koreans was particularly strong in late 1950s to early 1960s (Showa 30–40). Not only was a bank loan not possible but obtaining employment typical for a Japanese was difficult for Korean. Zainichi Koreans did not have steady jobs and were in a more difficult situation than Japanese. Many had a life of real "poverty and wandering." The total population of Zainichi Koreans in 1952 was 535,803 persons, among these, 61% were "jobless." In addition, among those employed, "daytime workers" comprised the largest proportion at 6.6%. Although the job category is listed as "commerce," most work involved "waste material collection" or working at eating establishments in stores such as at the military barracks and or selling makkori (Korean homemade fermented sake) and Horumonyaki (beef and pork grilled meat) in the Yamiichi (markets for trading based on a distinct illegally established market economy principle, in which prices were uncontrolled and which operated illegally when supplies were in short supply under the controlled price system).

Moreover, Zainichi Koreans were discriminated against regarding marriage. Mr. D recalls the following incident.

"When I was an elementary school student in the late 1950s, an old woman who lived in our neighborhood was wearing a white jeogori (Traditional Korean women's wear) and crying. When I approach, I could see she was burning a pile of clothes and crying so much. After I got older, I asked one of my brothers. He told me that her granddaughter was in love with a Japanese but couldn't get married, so the girl drank some chemicals and died. I don't know if it was ammonia placed inside a rubber ball or what. But I remember that. She was crying so much."

Zainichi Koreans were living a life of suffering.

4.4.2 Experiences in school education and formation of a negative identity

Not many Zainichi Korean children were enrolled at Mr. D's elementary school. But there were at least two or three Zainichi Korean children. During elementary school, Mr. D did not receive any daily harassment or bullying because he was Korean, but one thing happened when he was in the fourth grade.

Mr. D had good grades and was the class leader. One time, he got into a fight with another class leader over a trivial matter. They decided to "have a duel in the hallway" after school. All their classmates were watching from the classroom. The other child was big and kept kicking him, and they ended up grabbing each other. After the fight ended, the other child left shouting out, "Korean!" Mr. D was shocked by that word. He realized that "if I fight with someone, that is what they'll say."

"Even if we are friends, if we get into a fight, the other person will say that word. They've been holding it in for a long time. From that experience, I always tried to maintain a good relationship with others, as if everyone was my best friend. I think it cast a shadow on the development of my own personality and mentality. So, discrimination greatly influenced my personality formation. Of course, I'm not confident about a romance relationship with a Japanese, and I spent many dark days due to discrimination awareness. I wondered what was happening in my mental formation. In my first year at university, I had feelings of isolation while with fellow students. I thought this was 'because I am Korean.' I immediately noticed there was a thinking pattern connected to this. Do you understand this feeling? Discrimination awareness casts a large shadow on one's mental formation. As my own ethnic awareness was awakening, I considered how this affects and distorts one's mental formation especially during puberty."

Mr. D says that Zainichi Koreans face "discrimination" from the time they are young, and this largely influences the development of their personality and mentality. Instead of revealing his true self, Mr. D tried to be "everyone's friend" in order to avoid conflicts. All "Zainichi," especially second generation and after, have such experiences more or less.

Mr. D said, "I'm not confident about a romantic relationship with a Japanese. I spent many dark days due to discrimination awareness. I wondered what was happening in my mental formation." This demonstrates that he had questions and doubts about himself. Later, when he entered the university, he could get to know "fellow Zainichi students" and participate in ethnic related activities, which awakened his ethnic awareness. As a result, he could objectively view his own experiences since his childhood.

In the 1960s, Mr. D attended the same junior high school as children who went to Mr. D's elementary school and the neighboring elementary school. There were many Zainichi children in the neighboring elementary school. After entering junior high school, bullying and harassment of Korean children increased daily.

> "When I was going to M junior high school, it was very bad. It was in the 1960s. In history class, when the subject of 'Korea' arose, we would hang our heads. Children who attended school under their real names, which of course were different from Japanese names, were teased and bullied by the other students.
>
> I studied well for the first year. There were about 480 students in 10 classes in the same grade. 10 or 11 classes. Once, I was first in my grade. I attended school under my common Japanese name, and don't know where and how the other students found out, but a classmate who came from another elementary school said, 'Hey you, Korean! Board the ship from Niigata and go home!' That was so mean. Suddenly he came and said, 'Board the ship from Niigata and go home!'"

In the 1950s, there was a reparation campaign for Zainichi to return home to North Korea. On September 8, 1958, the 10th anniversary of the establishment of the Democratic People's Republic of Korea, Supreme Leader Kim Il-Sung said, "We sincerely wish to welcome the repatriation of Zainichi North

Koreans and guarantee all conditions." Since then, the General Association of Korean Residents in Japan started promotion activities targeting political agencies and local governments throughout Japan. From the Japan side as well, the "Cooperative for Zainichi Koreans Repatriation," was established in November by a nonpartisan group. In response to the expectation of repatriation, the General Association of Korean Residents in Japan supported North and South Korea's repeated advertisement as "paradise on earth." The Japanese government also quickly gave the "go" sign for this movement. Approximately 100,000 "Zainichi" took advantage of this repatriation to North Korea (Yang/ Yamada, 2014). The repatriation ships departed from Niigata. In other words, the words "Board the ship from Niigata and go home!" hurled by the Japanese child to the Korean children meant, "Board the ship and go back to North Korea."

> "There were nine teachers, but two looked down on Koreans in class. One was the history teacher and would say 'Korean' with a strange intonation. Another was the music teacher, and when everyone sung the wrong verse, he would say, 'it's in Korean' and everyone would laugh. Things like that. So, some of the classmates would say '〇〇kou' which I even hate hearing or saying. But they would casually say it."
>
> "One time I went home and cried, of course. My parents asked 'why you are ashamed of being a Korean?' From the time I was in elementary school, I learned things like 'the Korean peninsula was the route of Chinese culture,' 'it was just a bridge to transmit Chinese culture,' 'nothing is there,' and 'Japan ruled over Korea since the Yamato dynasty.' I only learned things like that. I kept hearing those things. That's why I felt so miserable. I spent many gloomy days. Since I studied, I somehow could go to high school. High school focused on preparation to enter the university, so everyone studied hard. I joined the sports club with three friends from the same junior high school. But soon quit. I stayed under the radar. For example, 'studying is meaningless,' 'even if I go to the university, it won't lead to anything.' It was a time when everyone was saying there was no work. I was making excuses. I couldn't concentrate on studying."

Regarding school education, speech and actions that were discriminatory against Zainichi Koreans was commonplace at the time. As a result, "Zainichi" children began to form negative viewpoints and ideas regarding "Korea," and "I am Korean." Mr. D went to a high school which prepared students to go to the university. In this environment, and since the path to career options was closed to "Zainichi," Mr. D gradually lost his enthusiasm to study.

4.4.3 *Continuing on to the university and the ethnic community*

Mr. D prepared for the university entrance exam for two years, and then entered a famous private university in Kansai. At that time, student movements were very active. Mr. D heard about the student activities at the university, such as "Communist/Anti-communist" and "All Campus Joint Struggle League" from his Japanese friends while preparing for university entrance.

Many young people were influenced by the conditions of the generation. He also had the experience that one student who had made discriminatory remarks to him in junior high school became a university student, and after becoming aware of social problems such as discrimination, apologized to Mr. D saying "Sorry about back then," when they met.

The student apologized saying "what I did was discriminatory. When I said 'Korean', I didn't mean it...I found that there was discrimination inside me." In that generation, slogans such as "No to the Vietnam war," "No to the Immigration Control Draft Law" were shouted.

His parents were very happy that he made it to the university. Mr. D was the only one among his brothers and sisters who went to a university. When he saw the examination results announcement and found out that he passed, he called home. His mother said "your father is very happy to hear that." His father said "I was also told that if I studied hard, I could go on to higher education. And with a scholarship, money wasn't a problem, but my parents didn't let me go." So, his father had an especially strong desire to be educated.

> "So, he must have been happy to know at least one of his children went to the university. Actually, he wanted to go on to higher education and study. When I was a child, father said his parents did not let him go to school, so he went and cried in front of the school. After graduating high school, he could have gone on to higher education under a scholarship, but his family did not allow it. It might have been because of the conditions of the generation. He said he could not go, so he went and cried in front of the school gate. So, he must have been so happy. Anyway, regardless of the resulting employment, my father could send a child to university, higher education. I took my father to my graduation ceremony. I'll talk about it later, but on the way home, we went to greet and thank the dormitory where I lived. After looking through the place, including my room, my father said to the dorm mother 'D still needs to suffer.' The dorm mother smiled and said, 'Mr. D's father, please don't make him suffer anymore.' As we walked from the dormitory to the station, he said 'you also suffered.' I looked at his face, tears were running down on his cheeks."

In the area where Mr. D went to the university, there was a dormitory for "Zainichi" students owned by a Zainichi Korean ethnic organization. The dormitory was nice three-story concrete building and had a large garden. Mr. D moved in during the fall of his freshman year. However, his parents didn't want him to move into the dormitory. They were happy he entered the university, but entering the dormitory also meant becoming involved in ethnic activities for Zainichi Koreans and political activities. His parents and brothers opposed saying, "you will be influenced by social activities," "you won't take care of parents, brothers, and family," "why do you work for the country while your family has so much debt and suffering." Despite their opposition, Mr. D left the house, and moved into the dormitory. He moved in because he was invited by senior students he met at the university who were also "Zainichi." He was obsessed and told his mother, "Please think that one of your sons has died." It became a humorous story to his dorm friends. But choosing to move into the dormitory led to much suffering for Mr. D. However, since he left the house and the family was poor, he couldn't pay the dorm expenses.

> "We were poor and at that time, the dormitory fee was several thousand yen per month, including breakfast and dinner. But I couldn't pay the several thousand yen. My university seniors said I could participate in the activities without worrying about the dormitory fee, but until one becomes a junior, part-time work is prohibited. I was receiving a scholarship from the Republic (North Korea) of several thousand yens."
>
> "I met a Zainichi student, and as my ethnic awareness gradually grew, I started to recognize that the discrimination in my experiences during puberty had cast a shadow on my mental development, and a fighting spirit emerged. The senior student said, 'Is it acceptable if our homeland cannot be united? This is a historical mission for us youth! Everyone, subjectively consider risking your life to accomplish this!' In other words, everyone was filled with this fighting spirit. It thoroughly permeated the dormitory, too. In September, I moved in as a freshman."

Mr. D's father used to be a board member of the ethnic organization S, which owns the dormitory. As a result, he saw many men, especially "Zainichi," become involved in ethnic and social activities, and neglect their family. Consequently, he worried that Mr. D would become "completely devoted to ethnic activities."

> "It seems that he was a board member, soon after the liberation. S was supporting North Korea, a socialist country. My father disliked the authoritarian frame of mind of South Korea. He hated it. But many people who were involved in the activities became activists and stopped caring for their family. Even persons in families suffering for poverty went to such kind of place and devoted themselves, even forgetting their parents and brothers. It was thought that if a son, even though he were poor, moved into a dormitory or similar, he would become 'red.' It was for that reason, not that he hated North Korea."

Mr. D's parents had special reasons to support North Korea. His parents came to Japan from Jeju Island. The Jeju Uprising occurred on Jeju Island in 1948. The Jeju Uprising was an armed uprising on April 3, 1948 by island residents who lived under the US ground-force command stationed in Korea and who opposed the independence election of South Korea. This led to the continued massacre of the island residents by the South Korea national police, South Korean army,

US forces, right-wing youth organizations, etc., until 1957. This series of incidents is said to have led to the death of 25,000–30,000 persons, approximately 10% of the island residents (Moon, 2005).

This included the death of Mr. D's maternal uncle and cousin. When he was a student, his mother told him that her brother's son went to the mountains on Jeju Island, perhaps for political activity. But everyone there was killed. Then their father became distraught and hung himself. Mr. D did not know that, having never seen either side of his grandparents. Mr. D has no recollection or fondness of his grandparents. With such historical background, his parents were never be able to accept the authoritarian government of South Korea. Until they died, their nationality was "North Korean." In addition, Mr. D's was a board member of S, a "Zainichi" ethnic organization which supported North Korea.

At Mr. D's university, a student Zainichi club would meet and engage in activities. The club was deeply connected to ethnic organization S' student organization. Mr. D was affiliated and involved in the club activities. On the other hand, Mr. D was very fond of Japanese chess. And his skills were very good. When Mr. D entered the university, he was considering joining both the Zainichi student club and Japanese chess club. When he asked one of his senior "Zainichi" students, the student advised him, "you just entered the university. Think about it after you get used to university life." However, while still undecided, his life became completely devoted to "Zainichi" club activities. In the fall of his freshman year, a "Zainichi" senior student found him playing Japanese chess at the Japanese chess club during the university festival. He angrily asked, "What are you doing? We are in a special situation!" In other words, "Zainichi" students in the club should learn about the circumstances of the Korean peninsula, their own country, contribute to the unification of North and South Korea, and put aside any personal hobbies. The place was tinted with the values that national and social problems should be prioritized over personal problems, and individuals should consider how to contribute to the nation and to society. At that time, the relationship between North and South Korea, and that between the Korean peninsula and Japan, was worse than today. With this generation in the background, Mr. D's campus life was centered only on club activities. "Although we struggled with discrimination in Japan, I was completely absorbed in the activities. Because I was a good student, when someone wanted to mention of a student from my prefecture, my name was the first to come to mind. So, I was really an exemplary student, even when I graduated. It was a long time ago."

4.4.4 *Work at the ethnic organization and onset of mental disease*

After graduating from the university, Mr. D worked full time at a company operated by the ethnic organization S.

> "As I expected, there was poverty and discrimination rooted in a person being 'Zainichi.' I worked so hard while at the university. When I was

graduated, all of the Korean graduates from all over Japan were gathered in the center. Then, assignments were handed out. I decided to transfer to the main headquarters of an umbrella organization. Normally, graduates become full-time workers of the local headquarters. I don't know if that was the policy at that time or not. So, right after I graduated the university, I became full-time worker at the headquarters. I say that because it was more than 40 years ago."

Mr. D received a small salary from the organization, including social and health insurance. He developed a mental disorder while paying his pension and is currently receiving a disability pension.

Onset of the mental disorder began in the mid-1970s, while working full-time. Mr. D did not explain the process in detail, saying that to do so would upset his future life. Instead, he said an "oppressive experience" caused the onset, as follows.

"There was an oppressive event. Since the source of unhappiness and suffering of the 'Zainichi' was the division of the fatherland, most of my fellow students considered democratization of South Korea and unification of the fatherland as their mission, and they studied and developed exercise activities.

I cannot talk about the process of onset of my mental disorder, but I attempted suicide, and there were various problems inside the organization. There is an unimaginable, unbelievable, unreasonable, and oppressive world.

I won't go into details, but as I look back on the world viewpoint 40 years ago when I was engaged activities as an activist, I thought personal advantage should not be placed above overall advantage. I couldn't separate protecting myself and personal egoism, and the thought of always discovering problems within myself. Something like that. As I continued to thinking, I noticed that my mental condition was like a slave. I thought I didn't understand the word 'dignity' or the meaning of 'human dignity.'

4.4.5 *Hospitalization and life under medical treatment*

Mr. D was accompanied by his older brother and admitted to the hospital. During consultation regarding hospital admission, his brother simply explained Mr. D's condition to the hospital director. The director asked Mr. D, "Do you want to die?" Mr. D was silent, thinking that whatever he said would just be a waste of time, and simply answered, "yes." He was then hospitalized in the closed ward.

"Once I was admitted, an iron door closed behind me, 'clang'. I thought, 'what?' There was a bed in a dark area to the side of the entrance. It looked like a bird cage. A man entered the cage, it was a very dark place, and administered an IV. There were two wide tatami rooms in the back, with 20 patients each. I wondered what kind of place it was and received a shot every day. It was difficult. Conditions were strange. The hospital itself did not have a good reputation."

The hospital stood out as a place that used dehumanizing treatment on its patients. Mr. D was discharged after one month of hospitalization. After discharge, he rested at home and waited for an opportunity. Since no one listened to Mr. D's claims, he went to work in Tokyo in the fall, and his salary was sent to him. There was an incident at work, which left him physically injured. He slowly lost his appetite. But he did not want to be hospitalized.

He knew it was related to his own mental disorder but thought he would surely die if he entered a psychiatric hospital like the previous one. He became emaciated and was told to go to the hospital, but he did not listen and he kept laying down at home. However, his condition reached the limit, and his father called an ambulance. He was taken to an internal medicine hospital over his objections. He was hospitalized for 10 days, but his condition did not improve, so he was transferred to another psychiatric hospital, different from the previous one. The new hospital knew how to handle patients. Mr. D said, "the nurses were good." Instead of force feeding him, they encouraged him to eat little by little, carefully monitoring his condition. As Mr. D started to think "Maybe I can eat," he gradually recovered his strength. When he was admitted to the hospital, his body weight was around 40 kg. He had lost nearly 30 kg.

He recovered to the point he could walk with the aid of a walker. "My parents were so happy, because they thought I would die. It was that kind of oppressive experience. I was there for three months, but finally I could eat and walk, and had gained some weight. I think my parents suffered so much."

4.4.6 *Conflict with a "left-wing activist"*

Mr. D was released from the hospital around the age of 30. Later, he was introduced to a company that manufactured household-use plastic by a former coworker and was hired. It was a sales job. He worked for a year and half. At first, he did various jobs, including office work, and while working at the company, he obtained a driver's license.

However, as Mr. D passed his 30s, he felt an emptiness regarding his job. The job was something to do temporarily, without accumulating anything. At the time, unemployment insurance could be received for up to a half year after quitting, so he thought it was an opportunity to acquire certification as a Labor and Social Security Attorney. He bought the textbook and studied by correspondence education and tried to acquire certification. However, he ran low on living expenses halfway through and eventually stopped without taking the exam, although he had applied for it.

Next, he worked as a truck driver, because he did not want to worry about his speech or deal with difficult human relationships like he had in sales. The company delivered newspaper to newsstands in national train stations at that time. There was a truck terminal in Osaka station, and his job was to deliver newspapers from the terminal to each station on the route.

There was a man working at the same place who also made deliveries, and was sometimes paired up with Mr. D. It was the early 1980s, and activities opposing construction at Narita Airport, which began in 1960s, were still underway. The man was involved in such opposition activities. According to him, he was in a sect and carrying out inter-group feuds. However, this is just what the man said, and Mr. D doesn't know if it was true.

The man was talking about the opposition activities to Mr. D during their delivery work. But Mr. D didn't want to hear such talk. For Mr. D, who experienced hardship due to political issues, the man's activities and what he was doing for work were entirely unrelated, and Mr. D did not want to listen to political issues.

Mr. D's biggest problem was "making money." His mother was old and sickly, and the charge for labor that his brother received from operating the machines had decreased and as a result, so did the family's income. Mr. D needed to make money for living. So, he worked hard. For him, this was the most important thing to do. In contrast with his thinking however, his coworker kept talking about political issues.

"The man 'came back from Narita' and sat down on the passenger's seat of the truck. Talking about 'Narita,' as I mentioned before, one of my friends who told me about a student movement while I was preparing to enter the university also said he went to Narita. He read a lot of books. The man at work talks to me about this and that. The way he talks is bad, criticizing the police, saying things like, 'killing a policeman, that's easy.' To see how much he studied, I mentioned the Marxist classics, just to see how much he knew."

"I won't criticize these activities anymore. As I look back, maybe he wanted to form an organization with me. Like, 'let's do it together.' But I had no intention whatsoever. So, when I said, 'I won't. My country's different,' he suddenly started to harass me. Something unbelievable happened that would disrupt my regular daily life. I don't want to talk about details, but the manager at work said that the man did the same thing to another employee who came from Okinawa. He was very angry at the man."

"The two-ton truck seated three passengers. Maybe it was just a coincidence, but there were iron pipes sitting on the passenger seat. Two short iron pipes about this long were sitting there on the small car seat. It was nerve-racking. So, I thought, 'That's enough! Why is this happening to me? I'm just a 'Zainichi' working hard at a company to earn money to live. This is too much.' I didn't try to get even, and I never said anything bad about him. I just said 'I won't do it.' Then there was the iron pipe. That was also nerve racking. I thought if something happened, this miserable life might end at the hands of this man."

Under such pressure and fatigue, Mr. D fell ill and was hospitalized again for several days.

After that, Mr. D started working at a company owned by a Zainichi Korean that traded with North Korea. Of course, North Korea and Japan didn't have diplomatic relations, but the relationship was not as strained back then as it is now. Private organizations such as trade delegations frequently came to Japan from North Korea. Many representatives of the trade companies from North Korea came to Japan and established "Zainichi" trade companies. Mr. D was employed at one of those "Zainichi" trading companies. His job was to respond to the trade delegations from North Korea. At one time, he often would hold conversations in Korean and could speak fluently to a certain degree. However, there was a long break where he did not speak Korean, and now he could not converse in Korean as he could before. He also felt a "difference in culture" and values between himself and North Koreans. The job became a burden, so after the probation month he quit. "During the second half, I became really sick. Due to the pressure, especially around truck delivery time, my head would hurt. As the days went by, I started to experience auditory hallucinations."

4.4.7 Recurrence and hospitalization

After that, Mr. D began to withdraw inside the house. His meager savings decreased. At that time, Mr. D was living in an apartment, but in his isolation, his condition worsened.

> "Gradually I didn't know what was going on. Sometimes I would roam around town in the middle of the night but couldn't visit my mother's house because she was ill. I was vaguely aware of my illness, and my sister told my oldest brother. He took me to the hospital in his car right away and I was admitted. I was in the hospital for four and a half years. As my condition stabilized, I thought, 'I need a place to work when I return to the area,' and started looking for work while I was still in the hospital. I didn't tell them I was in the hospital."

Because Mr. D wanted a job with the highest wage, he took another truck driving. However, when he started working, after arriving at the destination, he couldn't stand up when he got off the truck and fell to the ground. "I couldn't stand up correctly. I would jump off the truck and fall down. Even when I tried to get off normally, I would still fall. I was losing my balance. I would tumble like a ball. I couldn't stand up correctly, not even once. The driver never knew that the person from the passenger's seat was falling down. I would fall every time I got off the truck." That was his condition.

Mr. D lost confidence and hope in his own situation, and thought "I have become useless, I can't do any work," and quit.

> "I thought 'I'm hopeless. I can't be of use anymore.' I walked home around dusk. I felt miserable. As I was walking, I thought, 'I give up!' in resignation and sadness. There were times like that."

However, as he looks back, he thinks his loss of balance was due to regularly taking mood-stabilizing medication. Now the condition is indicated as a "side-effect" but at the time, such information was still not well known. As a result, Mr. D was disappointed at himself for being in such a condition.

"In desperation, 'I'm hopeless.' I was just going through the motions. I was in my 30s. I couldn't do anything, I just kept eating, exercise in the morning, eat, take drugs, then repeat. Even if I returned to my parent's house, there's nothing I could do. I couldn't work. So, I thought I would spend my whole life here and die. As I look back, I spent a meaningful life in my youth, but that's was it. I thought, 'I will end my life in this hospital. My life was really miserable.'"

"Then I was discharged, I guess the hospital provided guidance so that I would be released. I came out of the hospital four and a half years later. No one cared even if I returned to my parent's house, my old friends as well, even though I was in my late 30s. It was painful for me to go and see them. I sometimes hear various bits of good news about my old friends, but they didn't call me. Even if they did invite me out, I would feel miserable. No one came to visit me, and no one cared. I just stayed home, lonely and alone."

"I regularly visited the hospital for a year and a half. I didn't care, I would just receive my medicine, take it every day, each time. At that time, I gained about 20 kg, then 30 kg, after I was discharged, maybe because the medicine was changed before I was discharged. They always take a person's body weight at the hospital. Once a week. My body weight gradually increased just before being released. I used to be 60 kg or more, though. Every time my weight was measured, I would think I needed to reduce how much I was eating. I was in a room for eight people, I shared meals with the other patients in the same room, but I was still gaining weight. I gained 25–30 kg in one or two months after I was released. My body condition was poor because I suddenly gained a lot of weight. I've lost 20 kg since then and have gained about 10 kg from the time I was young."

4.4.8 Death in the family

Mr. D's father died at the age of 69 years in the 1980s. It was just 10 days after Mr. D started working in newspaper delivery.

"He used to sleep here. His heart condition was not good. Because this house was a factory, he would eat here and rented another place for the rest of the family to live. He slept separately. My mother and others could not sleep here. There was a space in between the machines at an angle, so he could lay a futon down to sleep. It was only my father and me on that day. We had a rental house nearby. I usually got on the last train of the night and went to the break room at the company. When I was leaving the house,

I checked the factory as usual. My father was sleeping, so I left him there without worrying. It was a chilly summer morning."

"I finished delivering the morning newspapers, and there was another morning lot that left around 8 o'clock. The truck was loaded with cargo and ready to leave. I was at the base of national railway with the bulk containers when a car from my company suddenly came up and said, 'Mr. D, your family called and said they want you to come back home right away.' Usually I would call back, and the family would say come home. I was going to say no. But when I called home, they said 'Father is dead.' On the way home, I didn't have any money, so I borrowed money from a coworker and got in a taxi near Osaka station. I was crying in the taxi and couldn't stop. The taxi driver asked, 'What happened, sir?' I couldn't stop crying. I was just wanted to start to be obedient to my parents. That was why I came back home."

"I thought, 'of course.' When I came to Tokyo, I thought I would be with my parents when they pass away. I thought, even if I was sleeping nearby, if I were a disobedient child, I wouldn't be there when my parents pass away. I kept crying then, at the funeral, and even now. I am right in the middle of poverty, while my brothers were also barely making a living, all with downcast faces. I was thin. It was hard, I cried and cried. I was crying all the time. It was really hard, anyways. After several days, there was a beer bottle. I drank from a cup which was next to it and felt better. So, I thought that's why liquor is on hand at funerals. I cried for days and felt a lot of pain. It was very difficult. I had a cup of beer after a few days. Then I felt better. It was a long time ago."

Then, in the early 1990s, Mr. D's eldest brother died.

"It was a day when no one cared. I had stockpiled drugs because I thought about dying. I thought there was no meaning to life. Then, all of a sudden, my eldest brother died. He died in his early 50s, when he was still young. I think poverty shortened his lifespan. Since my father died about 10 years ago, we always had a memorial service for him in the summer. One time, my brother said, 'Something is wrong. Why is my stomach so swollen? I will go to the hospital, after this memorial service is finished.'"

"My eldest brother had two children. The oldest daughter was outstanding, studied very hard, and was going to high school preparing to go to university. My father was very fond of her, especially because she was his first grandchild. My eldest brother was saying that she was a good student, and he was very proud, always saying that he wanted to send her to higher education, it didn't matter if she was a girl."

"The next child, his eldest son, was born disabled due to an accident at birth. Unlike today, there were few social services at the time, so my brother had to buy a car to pick them up and drop them off. We also did not have good understanding between us since we were children. When we would meet, we would just say 'it's difficult,' or 'because he has disabilities.' I was not sensitive in consideration of a parent's loneliness, sadness, and pleasure."

As a result, students of his home school decreased. Many cram schools were established, and since his only income was from the home school, his life was difficult. The charge for labor at the factory also decreased and didn't turn a profit. It was just enough to pay the equipment expenses. Working for free. My brother moved nearby but living costs were high. His first daughter studied hard, so he wanted her to go to a university. But his income is low. The factory didn't make much money, no one would fix the equipment when it broke down. My brother would quickly come and fix it. But he didn't receive any money. He didn't have enough for living expenses. So, he would work at the home school, and all night at the seafood market, then shuffle his son back and forth during the day. He had no time to sleep. He also ran a home school. Because his income was low. When I think about it, although I haven't seen his two children, I wonder how they are feeling, maybe sad and in pain."

"There was a Go club in the neighborhood. It was only 200 yen to play, so sometimes I would go there with a neighbor. Sometimes around 11pm or midnight I would see my eldest brother. 'Just drink a bit to relax. There's a place to sing karaoke which is very cheap.' I always would say. 'When do you sleep? You're going to die.' He really did die. He never got sick. He is the best brother- strong, filled with common sense, born before the war. He was well-built. He has had good social common sense. Whenever something happened, he did everything, he took me to the hospital. He was a good brother."

"My brother did not sleep at night. He had no time to sleep. Even I was telling him, 'you going to die.' When he said 'my stomach is swollen' and went to the hospital, he had cirrhosis of the liver. After I heard about that from another brother, he was admitted to a hospital near our house. In other words, it was too late. But I didn't understand that until later. If he improved, he would have gone to a bigger hospital. But he didn't, so he had to be cared for near our house in the end. It was cirrhosis of the liver. Every time I saw him, he had lost more weight, really. After he said 'I'm going to the hospital,' it was less than 2–3 months. He would lose more weight every time I went to see him. My mother wanted to visit him frequently because the hospital was near her house. Just to see his face. It must be difficult for his wife, too. Her own husband dying and unable to help. He was getting weaker and weaker. But I didn't want to believe that he was dying."

"One morning, my mother said she was going to go see him. I was saying, 'let's go there later, I'm tired,' but my younger sister, who worked at an office suddenly came in to the house saying, "Mom, brace yourself. He died.' My mother cried so much. It was so, really hard. I don't know how much hope she placed on him. But she didn't want him to die. Then when she heard, she cried "woah!" I never saw her like that. She cried so much. Her strongest and good son died. When I saw her, her whole body was crying and crying.

I thought that when a child dies before his or her parents, it would be like this. At the time, I was saving drugs, thinking there was no meaning to life. But I thought, at least, I should not die before my parents. That was why I kept living. If a child dies before his or her parents, it will be like this. After my emotions calmed, and I looked back on this a few years later, I wonder if she cried that much when my father, her husband, died. I thought that when a child dies before his or her parents, it would be like this."

In December of the following year, his mother died at the age of 81 years.

"It was another terrible story. She died at O hospital in early 1990s. O hospital took good care of her. She often had a high fever. After an examination, a young Zainichi doctor said 'we finally figured it out. It's biliary stones. Little stones had clogged the bile duct, that's why she has high fever.' She was 80, but the doctor said, 'she will be fine after an operation, if I remove the stones.' But my mother said, 'no, I don't want to.' She was 80 years old. Another man in his 40s had surgery by the same doctor, He said, 'I was cured by surgery and it went without any problems, but it hurts. When the anesthetics wear off, the pain is excruciating.' After we heard that, my brother also thought 'She's 80, but if the surgery is successful, she could live for another 10 years.' My mother kept saying no, but we strongly recommended it, so she said 'I'll try.' After the surgery, she had so much pain after the anesthetic wore off. The pain was extraordinary. I kept seeing her, hoping she would get better. I stayed over, I even worked at the factory. I thought she would be okay. If only she could overcome the pain. I went there all the time. But the sutures didn't stay closed. A month later, the doctor said 'I am going to remove the sutures.' He went into operation room then came out, saying, 'her intestines are sticking out, so I will perform surgery again.' The Zainichi doctor said. I won't forget his name. Then he went in, made an incision and performed surgery again. A few days passed. Do you think an 80-year-old person can survive two surgeries? She died. If she were to die anyway, we shouldn't have allowed her to have the surgery. We had no idea of a second opinion, and just followed anything the doctor said. She had a serious wound and died in pain. Do you know of such a son? I can never apologize enough."

"I told an old Zainichi medical person who knew my mother that she died. The person seemed surprised and sadly said, 'Operating on such an old person is unbelievable. The doctor just wanted to gain experience.' Oh, that doctor. Since my mother was receiving welfare, 'he could receive a large medical fee too.' That's what the person said. 'He is a young Zainichi doctor who wanted to gain experience.'"

"He didn't show up when my mother was on her deathbed. He had another doctor come. There was nothing we could do, just let her die in pain and suffering. I went to see him later. I couldn't accept how my mother died. I was not connected to anyone in the world and was going to the factory to work a side job for 90 yen per hour, I was going there with wearing sandals. I asked, 'why did my mother die?' 'Because your mother had a thick layer of fat. You know, the sumo wrestler Tamanoumi also died of appendicitis.' That was his answer. He doesn't say anything like 'I'm sorry.' 'Tamanoumi also died of appendicitis, because he had a thick layer of fat.' He never said he was sorry. Now as I think about it, my head was unclear. I had no mental strength or anything. If it happened now, I would hit him. Really. I would say 'Curse you! Call the police if you want. Go to police, curse you!' She gave a birth to me, raised me, and always protected me even when I was sick and difficult. She was my precious Omni, who loved me, right? I would hit the man, definitely. I am a pitiful son."

"Things like that happened, so I felt miserable. It was when I was released from the hospital and thinking, 'There is no meaning to life.' I wasn't connected to anyone. And no one cared. I was snubbed, and I personally did not have any confidence. I had a miserable life."

4.4.9 *"Tying multiple layers of vertical and horizontal threads together"*

The year after his eldest brother died, his mother died. Mr. D spent every day feeling like "there is no meaning to life." However, while his mother was alive, his younger brother who married to a Japanese woman would visit her every month, along with his daughters, his mother's granddaughters. While his mother was alive, she looked forward to seeing her granddaughters who visited once a month.

At the time, Mr. D was hopeless, with nowhere to go. He stayed home, always sleeping in his pajamas, while his mother and his younger brother's family were talking and laughing in the next room.

Those granddaughters grew and became elementary school students. Then, he said, "I thought I should not die while my mother is alive. Then, after my mother died, I thought that if these girls found out their uncle died under suspicious circumstances, it will be a burden in their hearts. I was just going through the motions, but more dead than alive."

In 2005, Mr. D changed his nationality from "North Korea" to "South Korea". Up to then, everything was North Korean, however, since he had the opportunity to organize his family registry of his own country, such as notification of death of his parents and brother, he changed his nationality and obtained a South Korean passport. In October 2006, he visited South Korea for the first time by an invitation from an NPO that provided support to persons with mental disorders. He had just started to participate in the activities of the NPO and attended a world conference in Seoul. "I went to South Korea for the first time in my life. The first time in my life. I never thought I would go to my mother country. I cried a lot."

At the same time as the NPO activities, Mr. D regularly went to a factory where persons with disabilities worked. By engaging in these social activities, he could gradually increase his friends. He used to say "no one cared. It was painful for me to go and see old friends and hear good news about them, but they wouldn't call me. Even if I go see them, I would just feel miserable. They all have their own life and are busy, and they have varying circumstances. Or maybe they don't know. No one came to visit me, and no one cares."

Mr. D spent many lonely days and knows such feelings of loneliness. He returns all of the New Year's greeting cards, and currently has more than 400 contacts, including many acquaintances in his cell phone contact list.

"I started to keep these things precious, and see their heart, no matter what kind of position they are in. Before their business title and ability, I see what is in the root of their heart. While looking at myself as well. Living with humanity, 'courtesy' as a human, especially 'trust.' I have determined to value my connection with these people. It is something I have deeply learned myself. Step by step. Before there was only one thread, the thread of isolation. So, I weaved multiple layers of vertical and horizontal threads together, no matter if one or two were cut, no matter what happened. It makes it easier for others to trust you if you are being yourself and your way of life is constant. That's the lesson I learned. Now, regarding layers. I have lived for some 60 years and learned many things. Now I think I want to live like a human, although it is quite ordinary. I would like to live the life I was given, thinking and considering 'what is the way of life as a human?', 'Am I living like a human?', 'What is it like to live with respect of oneself?', 'Am I doing it?' I sometimes will review myself."

Mr. D enjoys "Shogi" (Japanese chess) and "Go" which he has played since he was young. He holds the rank "dan" in Shogi and Go. He also regularly goes to a Tai Chi club. He says, "Now, sleeping pills are for when I need them. I look at myself now, my life is really interesting. I now live a life I had never even dreamed of or could have imagined when I was in the hospital and thought my life was hopeless." Mr. D still lives in the house he grew up in, and the interview was carried out at his house.

5 Sociocultural factors of Zainichi Koreans with mental disorders

5.1 Hate speech and stress

One symbolic problem surrounding ethnic discrimination and racism today is hate speech. Hate speech can be considered as an inflammatory act to promote social discrimination which creates hostility and hate toward a certain individual or group, based on attributes such as race, ethnicity, gender, or sexual orientation.

In Japanese society, hate speech is mainly against Zainichi Koreans, and cases on the Internet, in street demonstrations, etc. have increased since 2009. Street demonstrations in Korean towns in Tokyo and Osaka have been frequently carried out, and videos of such demonstrations have been published on the Internet as well. During these demonstrations, words filled with hostility and hate toward Zainichi Koreans, such as "kill both good and bad Koreans!" are shouted. Also on the Internet, people of the so-called "Internet right-wing" have continued to use derogatory terms regarding Zainichi Koreans and write words filled with hostility and hate.

In December 2009, "Zaitokukai" ("Zainichi-Tokken-wo-Yurusanai-Shimin-no-kai," a citizen group against granting privileges to Koreans in Japan) carried out "hate acts." The incident involved more than a dozen members of Zaitokukai who gathered in front of the Kyoto Korean Daiichi Introductory School (term at that time) gate in Kyoto city, hurling abuse at the school, teachers, and children using loud speakers and interrupting classes for approximately one hour. The educational corporation, Kyoto Korean Academy, filed a suit against "Zaitokukai."

According to the judgment of the first and second instance, eight former members of Zaitokukai, repeatedly carried out propaganda activities voicing anger such as "Throw Korean schools out of Japan," "Cockroaches, maggots! Go back to the Korean Peninsula," over a loud speaker near Kyoto Korean Daiichi Introductory School located in Minami ward, Kyoto city in 2009–2010. A video taken of the propaganda activity was published on the Internet. An appeal hearing was held, at which the Supreme Court decided to dismiss the appeal by the Zaitokukai side. The judgment of first and second instance ordered the cessation of propaganda activities within 200 m of the school, and a compensation payment of approx. 12 million yen.

DOI: 10.4324/9781003177050-5

Due to the actions of "Zaitokukai," many children at the site became fearful and started to cry. Some became sensitive to noises and sounds during the class after the incident. Hate acts including hate speech inflict deep mental and psychological pain to those targeted.

Radicalization of the contents of street demonstrations and hate speech that floods the Internet tends to deviate from previous acts of discrimination. However, essentially these are the same, demonstrating the potential of hostility and hate toward Zainichi Koreans in Japanese society. A "Survey of actual conditions of discrimination against Zainichi Korean youth" was carried out to determine how hate speech, discriminatory treatment, and ostracism toward Zainichi Koreans in modern society are experienced, and how Zainichi Koreans receive such.

In this survey, responses to the question, "What did you think about hate speech?" included "I was shocked" at 78.2%, "Sad, frustrated" at 44.3%, "I felt angry" at 50.0%, and "I was scared" at 21.8%. Regarding the question "What else do you feel?" descriptions such as "I wonder why people write such things. I also worry that one day, I may not be able to live in this country," "I wonder why such reasoning goes unchallenged." "I am worried if there is no solution." "I believe it a little," "Why do they hate us?" "I thought these things could happen. This may look like an unusual situation, but it can easily occur if it is not brought to the surface. The number of people who are having a hard time have not decreased." "I can't stop thinking about why they do such things." "Their anonymity scares me."

Mr. C, who has a mental disorder and is "half Japanese, half Korean," and whose history has been inserted in Part 1, started to use the Internet around 2003.

He said "I was surprised to find so many entries about discrimination and tried to avoid them as much as possible. A few years later, as I was browsing websites and YouTube while net surfing, I felt the frequency of groups related to politics and producing hate speech had increased. I started to become paranoid as such verbal violence spread, even though these did not inflict direct damage to me. In my own experience, since I have paranoia and a severe handicap, the appearance of these groups and their hate speech causes nothing but fear for mental patients like me. Watching those videos doesn't affect healthy people, but if I see them, I would hyperventilate and my symptoms of depression would get worse. The psychiatrist instructed me not to watch such things."

Henderson and Sloan (2003) describe the effect of hate crimes as follows.

"The most difficult issue for victims of racial discrimination and hate crimes, and the most considered topic by mental health workers, is the degree to which these people view their own experience as an attack on their core identity." (omission) An attack to one's identity, which cannot be changed, deeply affects the thinking of racial and ethnic minorities, both towards themselves and the community, and their sense of being protected. (omission) Victims of racial discrimination and hate crimes are clearly different from other crime victims, not only because they feel they are targeted because of their race, but also because they are members of a social group which almost always draws an extremely negative fixed concept and impression."

In addition, Morooka (2013), from Henderson, et al., lists 1) continued emotional suffering, 2) self-doubt, 3) feelings of exclusion (self-awareness of being targeted as different from the norm, being a minority), and 4) blaming themselves, as common psychological effects suffered by the victims.

In Japan, the "Hate Speech Act" (official name "Act on the Promotion of Efforts to Eliminate Unfair Discriminatory Speech and Behavior against Persons Originating from Outside Japan") was enacted in May 2016. "The Hate Speech Act" defines hate speech as "intentional and unfair discriminatory acts which promote the exclusion of foreigners and their children in Japan from the local community, such as threatening harm to their lives, physical abuse, or inciting contempt for such ones." and indicates that "In recent years in Japan, unfair discriminatory acts which incite the expulsion of legal residents and their descendants from our regional society, because such persons came from a country or area located outside of the Japan, have been carried out. This has caused serious schisms in the local community and has forced foreign residents and their descendants to experience much pain." Consequently, this Act "does hereby declare that such unfair discriminatory acts are not acceptable." However, this law does not carry any penalty provisions or prohibitive regulations. Opinions that doubt its effectiveness have been submitted.

5.2 Discrimination leading to moral harassment

Sometimes I receive questions like "Is there still discrimination against Zainichi Koreans?" When asked, I reply, "Yes, Zainichi Koreans still often face discrimination when looking for work, seeking to get married and renting a house." However, this answer is problematic. "If I explain it this way, does it really convey what Zainichi experience and feel?"

During the time of first- and second-generation Zainichi, acts of discrimination were clearly noticeable. For example, during their childhood, schoolmates would throw small stones and rocks saying "Hey, Korean." Or if they went to play at a friend's house, they would be sent back home, with their friend saying, "my grandma said, 'that child is Korean, you should not play with him.'" Some teachers would say, "You don't need to take the class, go outside and play in the sand pit." If such things happened today, it would be a problem. However, conditions in modern days are a little different. Such acts are considered as "bullying" in school education, or "harassment" in the workplace.

But the question "Is there still discrimination against Zainichi Koreans?" really implies "Are you really being bullied?" or "are you really receiving harassment?" Can the person facing discrimination directly say, "yes, I am being bullied," or "yes, I am being harassed?"

The question "Is there still discrimination against Zainichi Koreans?" does not reveal violent characteristics the same as questions such as "Are you really being bullied?" or "Are you really being harassed?" because the person lacks "first person awareness." And, in the background of such question is "does bullying really exist?" the real meaning is "if you are really being bullied, provide evidence," that such exists. This can be considered as adding insult to injury to the person who has faced violence.

Dovidio and Gaertner (2004) indicate that the racism in modern society is "aversive racism." This differs from "old fashioned racists" who directly and clearly show discrimination. Acts by "aversive racists" show more flexibility and seem like a contradiction. What is "aversive racism?" Dovidio and Gaertner describe it as follows, with the example of Caucasians and African-Americans in the United States.

Modern cultural values are based on "a strong belief in justice," "a sense of right" and "racial equality," which are valued by most Caucasians. However, within their cognitive, motive, and sociocultural process lie prejudice between groups, and most white people have negative emotions and beliefs regarding African-Americans. But they are unaware of such and nonchalantly say, "We don't have prejudice" and try to separate themselves.

These negative emotions that aversive racists have toward African-Americans, do not appear with obvious hostility and hatred. Instead, their response includes "discomfort," "anxiety," "aversion," and "fear." In other words, when any pre-held indications that the person is an African-American are discovered, "feelings of dislike" toward such African-American appear.

In this way, aversive racism includes a more positive reaction toward Caucasians rather than a negative reaction to African-Americans. It reflects approval of the ingroup rather than negative feelings toward the outgroup. It is used to clearly avoid the stigma of being narrow-minded, without damaging one's self-image of not being prejudiced. Aversive racists have racial ambivalence and show a fundamental double nature in their attitudes and belief. While showing racial discrimination that they can hardly avoid, they also wish to think "I am not prejudiced" at the same time. All forms of racism are not "aversive" or "tricky." Of course, old-fashioned racism still exists, and there are individual differences within aversive racism, and all Caucasians are not racists. However, aversive racism is still generally shown as a characteristic of the racial attitude of many Caucasians who like to think they are not prejudiced. And, under conditions involving racial issues or require contact between races, aversive racists show the following characteristics.

First, aversive racists support "just and equitable treatment," to every group, contrary to old-fashioned racists. Second, regardless of their conscience and good intentions, they are unconsciously uncomfortable with African-Americans, and consequently try to avoid contact between races. Third, when contact between races cannot be avoided, they experience anxiety and discomfort. Consequently, they try to separate themselves from the situation as soon as possible. Fourth, aversive racists strictly keep the rules of conduct and standards which have been set in situations where contact between races cannot be avoided because they have to act differently than they actually feel due to the fear that they may "appear to be prejudiced." Finally, they express their feelings by bestowing disadvantage to minorities, or provide benefit to the majority group in an unfair way by clever, random, and irrational methods (Dovidio & Gaertner, 2004). Does "aversive racism" correspond with the attitudes toward Zainichi Koreans in modern Japanese society?

In recent years, "harassment" occurring in various forms in the workplace, etc. has attracted attention. However, in the concept of this "harassment," there is the nuance that "what occurs involves one person to another." Japanese society tends to raise the topic of harassment so that it doesn't occur. On the other hand, however, the issue of "discrimination" is left to "smolder." Scenes that used to be recognized as "social discrimination" but which have now been consolidated into the concept of "harassment" are frequently seen. Social issues are intentionally changed to personal issues.

What is the difference between "discrimination" and "harassment?" The difference between "bullying" and "social bullying" should be understood as a problem between "one person to another," and as "society (majority) to an individual (minority)."

In modern times, do children who are bullies throw rocks at the children who are bullied so that others obviously know? Bullying sometimes occurs that way. However, in modern society, it is more characteristic for bullying to be carried out in a way that a person "can't grab the fox's tail" (not easily caught) rather than in a way that is clearly visible. This is bullying in modern times. In other words, modern bullying is "invisible bullying." This is the same with "discrimination." "Discrimination" in modern society is "invisible discrimination" in many cases.

Zainichi Koreans for example, since they are a minority, "are being silently excluded from within a group, isolated," "information is shared between members of the group, but not transmitted to a person who is a minority," "ignored," etc. Such "exclusion," "ostracism," and "disfavor," is the "discrimination" of modern society. So, can one really say discrimination has improved compared to before? Even though the style of bullying and harassment has changed, the victims who receive such still receive much mental stress and damage. As a result, they suffer mental disorders and commit suicide.

Regarding bullying and discrimination in modern society, it is more difficult for a perpetrator to have self-responsibility awareness. Acts that can be easily and objectively understood, such as throwing rocks, beating, and wild talk, can be more easily recognized by both the perpetrator and the victim. However, regarding acts that are objectively difficult to understand, such as exclusion, ostracism, disfavor, it is more difficult for the perpetrator to accept self-responsibility. True "aversive discrimination" involves bullying and discrimination, while maintaining the self-impression that "I'm not doing anything unjust or vicious." Consequently, it is easier to give the explanation, "I didn't do anything," or "I was just kidding." Perpetrators with poor self-responsibility awareness repeat the same acts. Persons who bully and harass others repeat the same actions over and over. Because they fail to realize how serious it is for the other party. Discrimination is the same. A characteristic of a victim of discrimination is being a member of a social group that one has no control over but is born into. The perpetrator does not realize how much his acts of exclusion, ostracism, and disfavor cause mental stress and damage to the other person, or how serious it is. On the other hand, they may do so with full awareness of the mental stress and damage suffered by the other person. Do they do those things in order to cause mental damage?

So the question "Is there still discrimination against Koreans?" is the same as asking "Are you really being bullied?" How can children prove that they are being bullied? The complaint, "I'm the only one being ignored. They don't talk to me," is invisible bullying. It is difficult to show proof. "Visible bullying" can be seen, such as "he/she said wild talk such as this," or "He hit me." However, bullying is actually done when others are not watching. Discrimination is the same.

In recent years, the term "moral harassment" has emerged. Moral harassment is unseen violence and is called "mental violence" and "mental domestic violence." With the spread of this term, more people have come to understand that denying "individual freedom/way of life" and not recognizing a person as an individual, is violence toward one's personality and violence that attacks the core of person's life (Megumi Tanimoto, 2012). Moral harassment is not just a problem of one person to another, but a structural problem that causes harassment or promotes its continuation. However, it is hard to see the structure. Discrimination in modern society is "aversive," and leads to "moral harassment."

5.3 Racism and stress

Many Japanese do not know what kind of people Zainichi Koreans are. If they are older, Zainichi Koreans must have been present in their daily life. And many people have actually had dealings with Zainichi Koreans as a real-life experience. However, younger people may not have the opportunity to develop a specific image of what kind of people Zainichi Koreans are. This may be due to Zainichi Koreans not identifying their own ethnic origins in many cases, and most Zainichi Koreans with North or South Korean nationality are in an international marriage. And it is common for their children not to inherit North/South Korean nationality. Persons obtaining Japanese nationality have increased and an objective indicator of who are ethnically "South Korean," or "North Korean" has become blurred.

It is also true that fewer Japanese have had dealings with Zainichi Koreans as a specific and actual experience. There is always the question, "Who are 'Zainichi Koreans?" Without experience, this can easily become an abstract image, and images become prejudice and preconceptions which are often spread through

Japanese society. As previously shown, this becomes evident as social distancing measures.

Prejudice and preconceptions of Zainichi Koreans are based on stereotypes. What causes some people to be stereotyped? It is the application of a specific characteristic shared by the majority or all members of the same group to certain people (Brown, 2010). And stereotypes are based on racism.

As a more comprehensive definition, racism can be defined as beliefs, attitudes, and established systems, including acts that tend to denigrate individuals or groups, based on biological appearances caused by the interaction of genetics and the environment, or by the affiliation with an ethnic group. However, this is not just a problem of the relationship between the oppressor and oppressed, but also includes racism between members of different ethnic groups, and the beliefs, attitudes, and systems that are established and perpetuated by racism in the group of the same ethnicity (Laveist & Isaac, 2013 ed.).

Such racism is a severe stressor that is often experienced by many racial and ethnic minority group members (Loue & Sajatovic, 2010 ed.).

> Experiencing racial or ethnic discrimination is one of the main causes of stress for many racial and ethnic minority women. Individuals face racism and discrimination in interpersonal, collective, and social activities, and in the political context. Sometimes, the stress is severe and chronic. When a stressor related to race is recognized as a burden on personal or collective resources, or overshadows or threatens a person's happiness, a negative result occurs. Mental pain and mental illness, including depressive syndrome, are related to stress, racism, and discrimination. Racism is a critical stressor which is often experienced by members of racial and ethnic minority groups. In contrast to the negative effect of racism is colonization, which includes important variables which act and influence on how persons bear and manage stressors. As a mediator of results, focusing efforts that support the mental health of individual personalities, in order to draw a blueprint, is important. Negative psychological influences of racism require continued attention.
>
> (Loue & Sajatovic, 2010 ed.)

5.4 Minority and mental disorders

The relationship between race and mental health is very complex. Breslau, et al. (2006) and Bratter and Eschbach (2005) report that the prevalence of mental disorders and mental suffering in African-Americans is lower than that for Caucasians and other minorities. On the other hand, Williams and Harris-Reid (1999) and Husaini, et al. (2002) report that the prevalence of mental disorders and mental suffering in African-Americans is higher than that for Caucasians and other minorities. In addition, according to Harris, et al. (2005), 21% of native Americans and Alaskan natives have some kind of mental problem such as mental disorder, and according to Duran, et al. (2004) and Fingerhut and MaKue (1992), they have higher suicide rate and alcohol dependency than Caucasians and other minority groups. However, differences in the mental health statistics between ethnic groups have shown a decreasing tendency. For example, among Asian-Americans, feelings of self-esteem are more strongly connected to occupational and educational indicators of SES (social economic status) than to income. These studies indicate that some groups are more susceptible to the influence of chronic stressors (for example, poverty, chronic disease, not married) which are commonly found in lower socioeconomic classes. The mental health of racial and ethnic groups is considered to be influenced by multiple factors (Stepleman, et al. 2010).

Cantor-Graae, et al. (2005) analyzed articles with the keywords "migration," "ethnicity," and "race," published between 1977 and 2003, and calculated the relative risk of onset of schizophrenia in first and second generation of immigrants compared to native residents, and then considered articles which did not separate first- and second-generation immigrants. The subsequent results were 2.7, 4.5, and 2.9, respectively. Incidence rate of schizophrenia over a person's lifetime was determined to be 0.85–1%. Cantor-Graae, et al. targeted representative items, "skin color of the immigrants," "social position," "uprootedness," and "discrimination" for consideration.

Moreover, Cockerham (2016) reported the current conditions of mental disorders in racial minorities in the United States in detail.

Accordingly, African-Americans comprised 13.1% of the total population in 2011. Kessler, et al. (1986), retrospectively analyzed survey data on mental health and determined that African-Americans are positioned in a "lower class" rank and suffer more mental pain than Caucasians. The authors indicated that these results suggest that the combined effect of poverty and racial discrimination inflict more pain to the African-American poverty group than the Caucasian poverty group.

In addition, Neff, et al. (1987) discovered that in Tennessee State, more patients with depression were African-American compared to Caucasian. It is more frequently observed that more African-Americans in rural areas suffered depression than African-Americans who live in urban areas and Caucasians who live in rural or urban areas.

In their retrospective study, Kessler, et al. (1999) pointed out "two main types of racism." African-Americans face daily discrimination in their lives. The "two types of racism" are "suffering at the hands of police," and the other is "being fired from work." 50% of African-Americans and 31% of Caucasians are reported to have experienced these, and mental pain and chronic depression symptoms were observed in both racial groups. 25% of African-Americans were daily aware of this discrimination, but only 3% of Caucasians did. Kessler, et al. do not claim that racial discrimination is directly connected to mental disorders, but indicated that such may cause psychological pain, and is more serious in cases involving mental health.

In addition, Takayama (2012) points out a strong dependency on alcohol, drugs, and gambling by African-Americans. He indicated that even though this condition is not "socially inherited, or a genetic or personality disorder," "they unavoidably face emotions of self-denial, such as 'I am not a good person.' This is unconsciously transmitted across generations. Regardless of how well you are living your life, you are denied by society. Even if you live as a citizen with a sound character, you are still discriminated against and are not accepted. If this is repeated, any person will lose confidence."

Next, Native Americans and Alaskan Natives comprised 1.7% of the total population in 2010 but had a higher rate of depressive disorder. The rate was approximately twice that for African-Americans, Hispanics, and Asians, and was also higher than that for Caucasians. This tendency can be seen in the results of numerous studies.

"Severe emotional issues" are generally observed in Native American children ages 5–8 years who live in a majority culture. And in young people between the ages of 10 and 20 years, "escalation of emotionally difficult issues and the use of drugs and alcohol" are observed more often than in Caucasian teenagers. The main cause of 75% of deaths and 80% of murders by Native Americans are related to alcohol. The second cause of death is "suicide."

In a survey in 2005, mortality rate by suicide in Native Americans and Alaskan Natives between the ages of 15 and 24 years, was 32.7 per 100,000 persons. This is approximately twice the rate for Caucasian males in the same age bracket. In addition, regarding the issue of suicide in Native Americans, further focus was given to young males.

According to Kamata (2009), Native Americans are a hotbed for serious alcohol dependency, due to isolation from the surrounding society, and a sense of stagnation and gloominess on an impoverished reservation. According to the US Public Health Service, the number of Native Americans who suffer from alcohol dependency is five times greater than the US average and mortality due to alcoholism is said to be seven times higher. A sense of stagnation, helplessness, and desperation is a deep-rooted cause. When one of the parents, or another family member suffers from alcoholism, the risk that the child will also suffer from alcoholism in the future is said to be twice as high. The negative chain continues within the household, and community values that were cultivated by tradition and lifestyle in the background are lost.

On the other hand, there are others with a different modality. For example, Hispanic-Americans, mainly comprised of Mexican-Americans, Cuban-Americans, and Puerto Ricans, have become the largest ethnic and racial minority in America, replacing African-Americans. In 2011, Hispanics occupied 16.7% of the entire US population. By 2060, they are estimated comprise approximately 1/3 of the entire US population, at 120 million.

According to most research resources, Hispanic-Americans do not show a high rate of mental disorders. Most studies on the mental health of Hispanics in the United States consider Mexican-Americans, as this is the largest Hispanic group. According to a study comparing Mexican-Americans to non-Hispanics, Mexican-Americans tend to have less mental anxiety. According to Burnam, et al. (1987), immigrants from Mexico to the United States tend to demonstrate a more positive degree of mental health.

Regarding characteristics observed in Mexican-Americans, they have a lower socioeconomic position and a higher level of "fatalism" than non-Hispanics. On the other hand, although fatalistic values and a low socioeconomic position in Mexican culture promote greater disparity, they tend to have strong family bonds which reduces anxiety. With this background, current studies indicate that Hispanic-Americans normally do not show a particularly high rate of mental disorders. In addition, this trend will not change with future generations, even in cases of low income, unemployment, inferior employment, poor housing, limited educational opportunities, preconceptions, discrimination, or language barrier.

Asian-Americans and Pacific Islanders also have very low rate of mental disorders. They occupied 5.1% of the entire US population in 2011. Asians and Pacific Islanders show a contrasting condition regarding mental health compared to other racial and ethnic minorities in the United States. Asian-Americans and Pacific Islanders have a higher income standard, education, and employment conditions, among minority groups in the United States and at times their level exceeds that of the Caucasian group. Furthermore, regarding mental health, Japanese-Americans have a very low rate of mental disorders. This can be considered to the influence of a very stable family structure and a strong connection with the Japanese community.

On the other hand, the number of Chinese-Americans admitted to psychiatric hospitals shows an increasing trend. In the background, a weakening of family and community bonds among the Chinese is considered to be a cause. Even still, the rate of mental disorders in Asian-Americans and Pacific Islanders is lower than other racial and ethnic minorities or Caucasians.

Up to this point, the condition of mental disorder among racial and ethnic minorities in America has mainly been considered, and based on Cockerham (2016), various differences between minorities were pointed out and are dependent on the history and situation of each group.

5.5 Zainichi Korean as an involuntary minority

Ogbu classified minority groups as "voluntary minorities" and "involuntary minorities" based on the differences in the process of joining the host society. "Voluntary minorities" are persons who move to a society believing it will lead to a better economic condition or more political freedom. They do not consider acceptance of the system of the host society and its treatment as forced or oppressive but tend to accept it as a task to overcome for personal and social success. For example, refugees, immigrants, and foreign workers can be mentioned.

In contrast, "involuntary minorities" are persons who are brought into the society through slavery, subjugation, or colonization. In many cases, feelings of resentment due to lost freedom, and that the system of the host society and its treatment toward them shows unfair discrimination and oppression. For example, the experiences of African-Americans and Native Americans can be mentioned (Nabeshima, 1993).

According to Ogbu's typology, Zainichi Koreans are involuntary minorities, but newcomer Koreans can be considered as voluntary minorities. Among "persons with North/South Korean nationality," "minorities" and "persons who experienced discrimination" have a higher rate of suicide, as indicated by WHO, are considered to mainly correspond to Zainichi Koreans. And from this viewpoint, the high suicide rate of "people with North/South Korean nationality." is considered to be influenced by Zainichi Koreans. However, another factor that should be considered is that Zainichi Koreans who have obtained Japanese nationality are not included in "people with North/South Korean nationality." If the suicide rate of Zainichi Koreans who have obtained Japanese nationality is included, the figures may be even higher.

Ogbu and Herbert (1998) stated that for minorities, this "voluntary" and "involuntary" presents a structure to recognize one's own conditions from a different viewpoint (status frame of reference). In other words, "voluntary" has two positive viewpoints. The first viewpoint is to reference their conditions within the host society, and the second viewpoint is to see their own conditions in reference to their homeland or mother country. Since they can frequently talk about their own success in the society where they moved to their family, they can accept their condition positively by these two viewpoints without contradiction or conflict.

In contrast "involuntary" has two negative viewpoints. For example, in the case of African-Americans, their first viewpoint is based on their socioeconomic position in US society, and the other is through eyes that see the socioeconomic position of the white middle class in the United States. African-Americans recognize their socioeconomic position as lower than that of the middle class. They resent the fact that Caucasians have more opportunities that are not available to them, and do not believe that America "is a society where anyone can succeed if given the chance." Both "voluntary" and "involuntary" inherit this framework of awareness based on the collective experiences and memory beyond their generation.

Zainichi Koreans can be called involuntary minorities. They were directly or indirectly influenced by colonial policy and then came to Japan. And after that, they experienced prejudice and discrimination in the host society. In Mr. A's history, his father strongly resented his own circumstances.

The effect on mental health greatly differs depending on whether the social stressors are used as "encouragement for success," or as "promoting exclusion and oppression." This is a major factor in determining the likelihood of mental disorder within a minority group.

5.6 Experience of immigration and marginalization

Berry identified personal and psychological changes brought by contact with a different culture, such as those experienced by immigrants, as mental stress due to acculturation, and determined this to be "acculturative stress" (Berry, 2005). If acculturation goes smoothly at the personal level, the person can be adopted into society. But when things do not go right, acculturative stress occurs, mental health is damaged, and symptoms such as depression are observed (Lee & Tanaka, 2011).

Four attitudes regarding this acculturation are "assimilation," "separation," "integration," and "marginalization." "Assimilation" seeks to live one's daily life immersed in the dominant culture, rather than maintaining one's own cultural identity. "Separation" seeks to try to maintain one's own cultural identity and avoid participating in the dominant culture. "Integration" seeks to participating to dominant culture while maintaining one's own cultural identity. And "marginalization" is when one does not (or cannot) maintain one's own cultural identity and is forced into cultural deprivation and does not (or cannot) participate in the dominant culture due to reasons such as exclusion and discrimination (Berry, 2008). In many cases of "marginalization," cultural inheritance is frequently lost, dysfunction and deviant behavior occur, resulting in antisocial behavior and dysfunctional family conditions (Berry, 2005). Mr. A's family was isolated from the Zainichi Korean community and did not have interaction with Japanese residents in the local community. Mr. B and Mr. C lived in an environment comprised only of Japanese and did not have opportunity to contact the ethnic community. For Mr. C, the branch chief of an ethnic organization was the first "Zainichi North/ South Korean" he met. So from this, all three were "marginalized." However, dysfunctional conditions in the family can also be said to apply.

5.7 Discrimination and trauma

Previously, the hypothesis that racism and discrimination in the modern society are "aversive," was introduced. Although not blatantly open as they were in the past, discrimination can still occur while adopting "equality" outwardly, while holding aversive emotions toward others and minorities, and still appears in certain situations.

Regarding "trauma," Miyaji (2005) focuses on "trauma of minorities." She says, while there are "extreme experiences as a human, such as war, concentration camps, sexual violence, trauma-like experiences," "there are also many conditions in the world, in which each seems very trivial. However, these chip away at the existence of the person, and eat away at the person's dignity and self-affirmation, for example, being of an ethnic minority held under colonial domination, receiving constant prejudice and discrimination due to various reasons, such as disease or mental disorder, gender, sexual orientation, etc. Although not visible like blatant violence such as cutting someone with a knife, there is still oppression and violence that is more chronic and is like slowly strangling someone with a silk cord."

In the field of psychiatric medicine and psychology, "trauma" is "damage by an unexpected catastrophic experience accompanied with crisis of life, whether physical or mental." In Japan, it is often used in the same way as the experience of emotional trauma. This trauma can largely be divided into "single trauma" which is experienced as a personal life crisis or that of someone close, such as war (terrorism), disaster, accident, or being a crime victim, and "complex (accumu-lated) trauma" which are repeated daily in the living environment, such as abuse or neglect" (Kato, et al. 2011). It is "the condition of being shocked by a past event which cannot be forgiven, and continues to cause fear and discomfort, and continues to influence the person even now" (Miyaji, 2013).

"Single trauma" is generally called as "trauma type I," and "complex (accu-mulated) trauma" is called as "trauma type II." Miyaji also mentions the concept of "trauma type III," where "a minority experiences traumatic events which seem small, but erode a person's existence over a long period, a 'silk cord type' trauma experience" (Miyaji, 2005).

I also think that when minorities experience contempt, discrimination, and experiences such as "passing" as introduced later, the possibility of a minority developing trauma is created. For minorities, such experiences happen daily and are accumulated over a long time. Consequently, they are harder to identify. However, a minority accumulates stress and mental and psychological damage from these experiences.

Persons in the majority who demonstrate "aversive racism," want to believe that they are persons who value equality and do not want to recognize that they discriminate against others, even though they target others for aversion. In this case, what does the majority do? The majority inflicts a "negative attack." While it is difficult for them to clearly admit that they show discrimination and oppres-sion, they still practice such by methods such as "ignore," "a quick glance," and "ostracism."

The majority direct judgment to the minority. "They are short tempered," "easily get angry," "are always upset," "constantly confrontational" … If minor-ities are short-tempered, easily get angry, are always upset, and confrontational, don't they deserve such treatment? However, this reasoning boils down to "self-justification."

"Basically, there are very few research surveys on the frequency of trauma in minorities in Japan," Miyaji points out.

> The suffering of minorities is hard to see by the majority side and is not well-known, so it is hard to be interested. Even if it is known, it can easily be viewed as "a specific issue" and not related to the majority.
>
> There is also taboo awareness. It comes from both sides. The majority wish to avoid topics which bring awareness to their own characteristics as perpetrator, refrain from talking about it if not a concerned party, worry about being criticized for saying the wrong thing, and afraid that such talk is viewed as political. On the minority side, they worry that, by bringing attention to the subject, they risk being discovered as a minority, that their aversion is just their own impression which is colored by the minority, and fear being criticized that they are absorbed in victim awareness.
>
> (Miyaji, 2013)

The discrimination experience itself is a trauma for the minority.

5.8 Socioeconomic factors

Another common background of the four people interviewed was the issue of "poverty." All the families suffered economically, and this led to dysfunction within the family.

In Mr. A's household, the father was an alcoholic and gambler, leading to domestic violence. Mr. A's mother regretted marrying him. Mr. B's father also had an issue with domestic violence, and Mr. B lived under oppressive conditions. Mr. C also experienced poverty, because his father died when he was a child and his mother had to support the family by herself. In addition, Mr. D's family had difficulty maintaining stable work because they are "Zainichi." They were always "working to pay back debts."

Mr. A's mother always told Mr. A "not to be like your father." On the other hand, when she scolded, she blamed him saying, "you're just like your father." Mr. B also had similar experiences. When Mr. B's mother scolded him, she blamed him saying, "you get that from your father."

Although domestic violence is the norm, it should never be forgiven. However, the problem will not be solved simply by the essentialism. Turning attention to socially constructive aspects is also needed, right?

Lee and DeVos, et al. (1982) carried out an interview survey in the late 1970s and reported that a characteristic of Zainichi Korean households is "the wife despises her husband." Zainichi Koreans in Japanese society suffer discriminatory treatment in their daily life, and at important moments in their lives, such as employment and marriage. Men are specially excluded from opportunities to gain stable work that matches their abilities and qualities due to discriminatory treatment. While Japanese men of the same age were employed in stable jobs, Zainichi Korean men were employed in unstable jobs and under severe labor conditions.

The society of the Korean peninsula has stronger Confucian thinking than Japan. In the world of first- and second-generation Zainichi, Confucian ethics, and rules are deeply reflected in their life. The family was based on the patriarchal system, and fathers bore the role and responsibilities as the head of the family. It is not only the role to provide spiritual and normative support to the family, but also the role to ensure economic stability to the family. Through these responsibilities, the head of the family gains the family's respect as the head of the house. In many cases, however, Zainichi Korean men could not fulfill this role. As a result, wives and children thought, "even though all the Japanese fathers can receive a steady income and provide a stable family life for their family, why can't our father?" which leads to the evaluation that, "because our father is incapable." In turn, the fathers are aware of such evaluation, have their dignity bruised two ways – they are despised as Zainichi Korean in society, and they "lose authority as the head of the family." In turn, the father seeks to handle his stress through alcohol and violence toward the family, leading to dysfunction within the family.

Cockerham (2016), quoting Boardman et al. (2001) and Jackson (1997), stated that in consideration of their lower hierarchic rank, greater mental distress is observed in African-Americans compared to Caucasians. Mental issues are considered to be based more on socioeconomic factors rather than differences in race, etc. For example, the difference in the rate of mental disorder between African-Americans and Caucasians is normally considered to be caused by socioeconomic factors.

Generally, conditions related to stress and support are conversely related, increasing and decreasing in opposite directions according to social rank. So, as rank decreases, stress increases and support decreases. This is called systematic relativity (Kleinman, 1991–2012).

However, this does not mean that socioeconomic factors are the primary cause for the onset of stress and mental disorders, and racial and ethnic factors are secondary. In the formation of social rank, social discrimination caused by racial and ethnic factors are considered to lie in the background in many cases. It is easy to imagine that stigma caused by racial and ethnic factors makes minorities more susceptible to stress. The reason why racial and ethnic factors are not particularly sought in relation to the onset of mental disorders, is to avoid promoting racism through the stigma connected with mental disorders.

5.9 Stigma and passing

For Mr. B, "Korea" and "Korean" were "loathed and hated." In other words, for Mr. B, being a Korean was considered to be a "stigma."

"Stigma" as previously mentioned in detail, "draws attention to persons who would have otherwise been accepted under normal social negotiations, and forces them to look away, ignoring other favorable attributes," and "viewing the person as different from what was expected" (Goffman 1963–2001).

"Passing" refers to "how information about one's own weak point, when the specific problem is not immediately visible and is unknown to others (or at least the person doesn't think others know), is managed or handled. (omission) In other words, passing deals with the problem as to whether something should be shown to others or not, should they be informed or not, should the fact be hidden or not," and "how should such information be managed and handled with regard to those who would lose trust, even though it has not been exposed (or if it was exposed.)" (Goffman 1963–2001)

Passing seeks to identify oneself in relation to other people or to a group that is considered more favorable, not just by outwardly visible actions, but also from within a person. Among African-Americans, this is fundamentally found to occur in people who have mixed African blood with skin color comparatively close to Caucasians and is spoken of as a phenomenon to try to erase one's own racial origin and distance oneself from the disadvantageous condition as an African-American. This "passing" phenomenon is then applied to other people in other situations, becoming a completely normal cultural phenomenon and which thinking functions both socially and psychologically, regardless of the first principle among social rank, ethnic origin, or racial group (De Vos, et al., 1990).

Mr. B said, "I always worried about whether others would learn that I was Korean. I always appeared to be serious and gentle, and pretended to be Japanese." Mr. B would mark out the word "Korean" in his textbook and glue the pages together. "Korea" and "being Korean" were certainly a stigma for Mr. B. Behavior "pretending to be Japanese so others would not know" corresponds to passing.

Fanon states the following. "When a Negro comes in contact with the Caucasian's world, he has a certain hypersensitive reaction. If his mental composition is weak, it will lead to self-destruction. Black people stop acting as a proactive individual (actionnel). The purpose of this action is to become someone else (to become a white person). Only others can give him value" (Fanon 1951–1994).

However, passing comes at a cost. There is "loneliness and isolation" (De Vos 1992). Some people who do not choose passing feel repulsed by those who do choose it. In such case, persons who choose passing try to provide some kind of proof of loyalty to the minority group, and secretly try to associate with them. Devos stated that if a Zainichi Korean does not pursue passing, the person will actually pass through five phases, regardless of them being positive or negative.

First, in some cases, a setback in general achievements causes the person to recognize his lack of authority and rights. At times, this will lead to the pursuit of obtaining authority. At other times it will take the form of political expression and social resistance.

Second, there are some cases where success in a professional field or the business world within the collective Japanese society is achieved through one's own abilities. Such persons do not join an organization in general Japanese society or seek support. Many Zainichi Koreans have achieved success in the entertainment or sports world, or the restaurant business. Some of these individuals choose passing, and there are also cases where such persons have clearly stated their Korean identity.

Third, among the many Koreans who are socially excluded, there are some cases of criminal conduct. Koreans who have been comparatively successful in Japanese criminal organizations can be observed. Even in those cases, many are under passing conditions.

Fourth, in some cases, self-actualization comes to the surface in the form of ostracism or socially deviant acts. Behavior by "Zainichi" youth is manifest in a way that is difficult to be socially evaluated. These are acts of anger against that which is called "public authority," and is an expression of deep emotional or physical deprivation.

Fifth, difficulty in picturing one's own future vision is an issue, especially among youth. There are many conditions for social and psychological exclusion, and alcoholism among Zainichi Korean men is extremely high. General contempt for men also exists within families damaged by alcoholism. Contempt toward them in Japanese society leads them to drink, which in turn results in the loss of authority in the family as a father. In many cases feelings of self-contempt and lack of trust in one's own abilities are also manifest. In addition to economic deprivation, there is also emotional deprivation. This means that a "Zainichi" family is always vulnerable to social contempt against "Zainichi."

Kim Jang Su (2001) also mentions the adult-child syndrome mentality as a result of a dysfunctional family or alcohol dependency in the family, as an element of "Zainichi syndrome." However, the above indications were defined by De Vos in 1992, and the indications by Dr. Kim were defined in 2001. Both indications were made some time in the past, and applying these conditions to "Zainichi" under today's conditions may be considerably difficult. However, according to the experiences of "Zainichi" youth in the previously shown questionnaire survey and the high rate of suicide, it is reasonable to think that the conditions were not just in the past, but also exist today.

In any case, passing, as chosen by many Zainichi Koreans, forces a person to be nervous and that nervousness is not temporary but continues throughout their life. Actually, Mr. B also was told by his attending physician that "his tense feeling was greatly affected by his social environment where he must continually hide his ethnic origin." Passing affects minorities in this way.

5.10   Marginal man and multiple identities

The stance "marginalization" as presented by Berry has many points in common with the concept by Park and Stonequist many years ago, and the "Marginal Man" by Lewin (Park 1928; Stonequist 1937; Lewin 1948).

Ohashi (1980) also pointed it out and previously described that Zainichi Koreans can also be considered to have the characteristics of the Marginal Man. They are a minority that does not fully belong to either the culture of Japan or that of the Korean peninsula and have a fringe existence and marginality which exposes them to prejudice and discrimination in Japanese society. In addition, the relationship between Japan and the Korean peninsula is complicated by strong conflicting and nationalistic emotions due to historical developments and various political circumstances in modern society. Moreover, as shown in the results of the previous questionnaire survey, "South Korea" and "North Korea" are often targeted by Japanese society with repulsion and contempt. Under such conditions, Marginal Man characteristics can be attributed to Zainichi Koreans.

"Marginal Man" can also be called "a person on the border" or "on the fringes." According to Park, a marginal man is "a cultural mongrel who lives by closely relating to two different ethnic cultures and traditions. He does not voluntarily cut off himself off from his past and tradition, even though such is allowed. He is not fully accepted into the new society where he must newly create his own place due to racial prejudice." In other words, "a person who stand on the margin between two cultures and two societies which do not completely access each other or merge together." He is caught in "an ambivalent role where expectations are mixed and does not know which course to follow. In addition, his situation is one where he must change his behavior under certain conditions and act a different way under different conditions, depending on the values of those connected to the condition. This constantly occurs," and "he must stand between two representative and different cultures, and is caught between them, experiencing two conflicting cultures as his own inner struggle" (Orihara 1969).

Orihara described the characteristics of Park's "Marginal Man" in detail, and first mentions that Marginal Man's ego is divided in two based on the dualism of the world to which he belongs. It is divided between the ego formed as expected and demanded by one culture, and that of the other culture. Second, this division causes his actions to be inconsistent and unstable. At the same time, as his emotions must change each time he passes the border between the two worlds, he cannot avoid becoming unstable as well. Third, regardless of which world he is in, he easily attracts the attention of others. Especially in cases where a mixture of characteristics is outwardly shown, he is under the watchful eyes of others wherever he is. Since he is aware of "gazes," and "being watched by others," his attention is also drawn to himself. He becomes a person with strong self-awareness and regret. Fourth, when he wishes to adjust his attitude which changes each time he passes between the two worlds and tries to build a self-consistent and unique attitude, his ego is divided, and he experiences intense internal strain. Fifth, he cannot fully belong to either world, and to a certain extent, becomes a "foreigner" in both. As a result, his search for belonging is not satisfied, and he always feels uneasy because he is not standing on a firm ground, it is a "rootless plant" feeling. On the other hand, since the two cultures counter the grasp of the other, the particularities and relativity of both are found within the person and can be handled while maintaining a certain distance from either culture. Sixth, how he handles emotions changes depending on whether he is with other people or by himself. In a collective condition, he feels uncomfortable due to being aware of "gazes," is self-aware and nervous, and wants to quickly escape the situation. In contrast, when he is alone, he is affected by feelings of emptiness and loneliness as a wandering person, and his desire to belong increases.

In addition, people caught between Japan and North/South Korea, so-called "halfs" (double), are said to be people who were placed in a fringe position, even within the world of Zainichi Koreans, who are Marginal Man.

> When looking at 'doubles' from the social context, they can be viewed as 'doubly oppressed,' excluded and marginalized from both Japanese society and Zainichi Korean society. In other words, in Zainichi Korean society, they are viewed as 'impure' because of their mixed descent, while facing prejudice and discrimination in Japanese society as a "heterogeneous person.
> (Lee, 2016)

The category 'Zainichi Korean' is reproduced under a 'big story,' (=collective memory) such as 'multiculturalism' in Japanese society, and 'resistance' in Zainichi Korean society. 'Doubles' are 'doubly oppressed,' excluded and marginalized from this 'big story.' Many fall into identity crisis over the question of whether they are 'Japanese or Zainichi Korean?' due to the gaze into their heterogeneous and mixed characteristics and are negatively evaluated as a 'double.' In recent years however, people who overcome the struggle by affirmatively understanding and correcting 'double' characteristics, namely 'being Japanese and Zainichi Korean,' have appeared.

(Lee, 2008)

Furthermore, people with Japanese nationality are also placed in a fringe position in the Zainichi Korean world.

Koreans take a negative attitude toward people with Japanese nationality. If a person has Japanese nationality, and not North or South Korean nationality, he is not accepted as an official member of "Korean" community. People with North/South Korean nationality comprise the major portion of those in Zainichi Korean society, and interest in persons with Japanese nationality has waned. Like many "Japanese persons," those in Zainichi Korean society also can connect with North/South Korean nationality and their ethnicity as Koreans. Naturalization is viewed as a "betrayal," and naturalized people are viewed as persons who abandoned their Korean identity to become Japanese. In Zainichi Korean society, people with Japanese nationality have a marginalized existence, and are viewed as "semi-members" (Kashiwazaki, 2007).

Mr. C, who is "half" stated, "I felt like 'halfs' existed below 'Zainichi' society, something like 'an appendage.' I feel like 'halfs' appear only when convenient, such as bringing out a 'half' to promote the end of discrimination, something like 'let's aim for a society of coexistence.' I think Zainichi society is narrow-minded. I feel uncomfortable because I think 'Zainichi' talk about 'halfs' within the range of 'Zainichi society'."

In addition to being "half," Mr. C lives with multiple marginalities such as a sexual minority who is transgender and homosexual. In addition to his inner struggle and identity crisis as an ethnic "half," there is also his sexuality.

In cases where a person is a sexual minority, cases where his/her family are in the same condition are almost non-existent. In that sense, the person and his/her family have different attributes. In addition, it is common for the family to have preconceived ideas and prejudice toward sexual minorities. Hence, for a sexual minority to come out to his/her family is said to be more difficult than for people around them. There are many cases where, even if a person comes out, his family cannot accept it, and the person is rejected, ostracized, or excluded. Sexual minorities are isolated from both society and their family. In other words, they face "multiple isolation." Because of such a complicated situation, it is well known that sexual minorities have a higher rate of suicidal thoughts and suicide attempts than other people.

According to Harima and Ishimaru (2010), according to a survey on suicide-related occurrences by 1,138 people with gender identity disorder (GID), 62.0% experienced suicidal thought, 10.8% attempted suicide, 16.1% committed self-injury, and 7.9% experienced a drug overdose and these peaked when they reached puberty.

Although not a survey on GID, Hidaka et al. (2008) reported that the number of gay and bi-sexual men in Japan who attempt suicide (and fail) is approximately six times higher than that for heterosexual men. In addition, this survey also reported that among the 62% of total persons with suicidal thoughts, 57.1% were FTM (female to male), and 71.2% were MTF (male to female). Among those with suicidal thoughts, persons who actually attempted suicide were 10.8% of the total, 9.1% of FTM, 14.0% of MTF.

Regarding psychosocial factors leading to suicide, "bullying," "feelings of isolation," "physical dysphoria," "failed love," "internalized transphobia (various aversions to GID and transgenders= comment from the author)," "wish to reborn," "loss of reason to live and feeling of worthlessness," "obstacles in physical treatment," and "loss of hope in the future" are mentioned (Harima/ Ishimaru, 2010).

In the "proposal to review the comprehensive policy of suicide prevention (final plan)" published in 2012, by "the working group for the proposal to review the comprehensive policy of suicide prevention, National Center of Neurology and Psychiatry," "issues faced by social minorities" were raised as a point of focus for "each area of suicide prevention and recommended approaches." However, regarding social minorities, the only sexual minorities mentioned as follows:

> Regarding people with GID, gender dysphoria, and others who are subjected to social prejudice due to their sexual orientation (sexual minorities), the rate of psychological complications such as depression and neurosis is high, and suicidal thoughts are common. Suicidal thoughts often first peak during puberty when frustration due to physical changes caused by secondary sex characteristics, the issue of school uniforms in junior high school and issues regarding love overlap. As a response at the school level, providing information on GID and sexual orientation to parents and guardians and providing education to deepen understanding of the various genders of all the students, in order to promote the support of sexual minority children and further understanding in each household, as well as establishing a system where schools and specialized medical facilities can coordinate, are needed. Suicidal thoughts often peak a second time just before and/or after joining society, when difficulties in employment and issues regarding marriage are felt. In response, approaches such as training on human rights from the viewpoint of gender and sexuality, should be carried out at companies and the regional community in order to provide accurate knowledge and eliminate prejudice and misunderstandings.

Mr. C is a sexual minority, and "half" Japanese and Korean. He has multiple internal risks. However, he does not fit in the ethnic community world, nor in general society. Mr. C, with attributes such as "half Japanese, half Korean," "sexual minority," and "person with mental disorders," can be called "a minority among minorities," and "a double or triple Marginal Man."

Confirmation of ethnic bonds and ethnic identity was originally set as the primary goal of Zainichi Korean ethnic groups. Therefore, characteristics other than being "Zainichi Korean," such as, "a person with mental disorders," or "a sexual minority," are not subjects of positive discussion. Those characteristics are often treated as a local story (personal issue) in the ethnic world and are excluded from the dominant story (official history and description) of Zainichi Koreans, even if the person's social and historical background includes being a Zainichi Korean.

In recent years, addressing personal identity issues, not as a single element, for example, "only by ethnic identity," or "only by sexual identity," but rather as multi-layered and multiple elements, such as ethnicity, gender, and disability, has become common (Butler 1990–1999). Ignoring these multi-layered characteristics and the complexity of identity, and squeezing them into one, will have an oppressive function.

5.11 Regional community and isolation

Citing Cantor-Graae, et al. (2005), Noguchi (2008) explained the sociocultural factors leading to the onset of schizophrenia, as follows. The subsidiary position of African-Americans as outsiders who experience "social defeat" is assumed to be related to the high onset rate of schizophrenia in immigrants. In addition, the fact that second-generation immigrants have a higher onset rate than first-generation immigrants indicates a correlation with a disadvantageous environment. Unstable employment, poor living conditions, low social standing, prejudice, and racial discrimination can be described as a "disadvantageous environment." On the other hand, it has been reported that as the ratio of immigrants gathered in the region increases, onset becomes less noticeable among the immigrants. In other words, as the group becomes larger, it can act as a preventative against the onset of schizophrenia.

Similarly, Noguchi referred to a hypothesis by Halpern (1993) that African-Americans who later develop mental disorder, strongly pursue their goals and have a tendency to integrate into white society. On the other hand, they have a weaker sense of belonging to the African-American society, show an ambivalent attitude, and tend to separate themselves from African-American groups. As a result, they cannot receive support because there aren't any African-Americans around them. In addition, they more frequently face prejudice from Caucasians. Furthermore, although they seek to be successful in white society, they cannot achieve the things as hoped. As a result, people who are ambitious and have a weaker intention to integrate with African-Americans society, are at higher risk of developing a mental disorder.

In the course of the onset of a mental disorder, as connections with the surrounding society become diluted, individuals in lower social positions gradually develop lower self-evaluation because of their low social position. Even in such a disadvantageous environment, when these people live their lives in the region as a group, a protective effect of the collective becomes a strong vector to prevent onset. Of course, just gathering together people with the same circumstances is not enough. Helping one other and building a relationship of trust are also essential. At such time, although their circumstances may not be the best, they may not feel as unhappy. However, when an individual does not have a sense of belonging to the group he/she is affiliated with, the person stops having interaction with the group of his own initiative. Material and emotional support from the group is no longer received. In addition, they directly face prejudice and hostility toward minorities more frequently. These individuals ambitiously put forth great effort while denying their own origin. But in many cases, they cannot acquire or achieve their goal. This setback leads to the onset of mental disease.

In recent years, cases of Zainichi Koreans leaving ethnic residential areas to live scattered about in Japanese society have increased. Once busy regional communities have become areas where elderly people live, and where third, fourth, and later generations have left to live in "suburbs" centering around the Zainichi Korean community or become "buried" within Japanese society. In Zainichi Korean residential areas, the once cohesive property and unity as a group has weakened.

In the previous Zainichi Korean communities, there was mutual benefit to living shoulder to shoulder within the severe conditions of Japanese society. And this is how the communities were maintained. However, as years passed, the obvious discriminative treatment by the earlier Japanese society has decreased, and the option to obtain Japanese nationality has also become common. From this background, the socioeconomic low position of Zainichi Koreans has relatively dissolved compared to before. This has led to a decrease in the need for Zainichi Koreans to help each other, and as a result, the population of "Zainichi" who live in specific residential areas has also decreased. "Korean towns" where Zainichi Koreans used to live, have transformed into "ethnic towns" where newcomer Koreans and various races and ethnicities live. On the other hand, Zainichi Koreans who leave such residential areas and moved to live in Japanese society are isolated. In addition, people who live without identifying themselves as Zainichi Koreans have become part of the "majority." In other words, even though modern Zainichi Koreans are physically and mentally independent, their mental stress and feelings of isolation are thought to have increased, facilitating situations such as mental disorder and in the worst case, suicide.

5.12 Political nature and ethnic community of Zainichi Koreans

Mr. A came in contact with ethnic organization N and started to become aware of his own ethnic identity through the activities of the organization. And, while studying the history of Japan and Korean peninsula and Zainichi Koreans, he started to become aware of his own family environment, his father's experiences, such as dependency on alcohol and gambling, domestic violence, and his mother's experience and mental disorders such as depression caused by her relationship with his father, were not "personal issues" faced only by his family but were a "social issue" formed by the sociohistorical position of "Zainichi Koreans." This was also an opportunity for him to objectively review his own experiences and his relationship with his father and mother, and objectively understand the social factors related to the onset of his mental disorders.

The ethnic community was an opportunity for him to externalize his own development environment. However, for persons who were part of that organization, the existence of persons who were raised in an environment like Mr. A and who had mental disorders were from a "different world." Mr. A says, "Most of them were from ordinary families. All of them graduated from a university and were raised with no problems."

In that ethnic community, Mr. A hoped to "share with more people the causes that led him to develop a mental disorder, and the relationship between mental disorders and society." However, this was not realized, and Mr. A says, " I don't feel alienated, but I do feel a little bit lonely." The ethnic community for Mr. A was a place to share ethnic identity. However, his own existence with a mental disorder was not accepted, so it is considered to be ambiguous.

Confirmation of ethnic bonds and ethnic identity was originally set as the primary goal of Zainichi Korean ethnic groups. Therefore, characteristics other than "being Zainichi Korean" are placed in a marginal position.

Why did his father, a first generation of Zainichi, become an alcoholic and gambler, and show domestic violence? Mr. C is half Japanese, half Korean, and a sexual minority. As a result, he wondered "who am I?" However, "Zainichi society" did not respond to those issues. In the ethnic community world, the experiences of the four interviewed people can be understood as "personal issues." Mr. C felt such a "Zainichi" society was "narrow-minded," and the "Zainichi society" could be considered a factor of self-ostracism for him. Zainichi Korean society may no longer be relevant as the original meaning of "Zainichi Korean society."

Fordham and Ogbu (1986) drew attention to the "fictive kinship" in the African-American community as a factor in the low academic ability of African-American children. The concept of fictive kinship is used in the field of anthropology to indicate a "fictional family relationship." It is the "social and economic mutual relationship based on fictional connections which are not based on blood and marriage." In Japan, the relationship of "a midwife," "a godparent at the birth of a baby," and master and disciple relationship among craftsmen and in the traditional performing art world, can be raised as examples.

The fictive kinship in the African-American community "was formed as a way to compete in white society against the discriminatory experiences within the slave generation and after, and the stereotyping of the African-American experiences in white society. It is an awareness of the solidarity among African-Americans in white society and the collective identity which seeks to protect and maintain the borderline between Caucasians and African-Americans" (Fordham & Ogbu 1986; Fordham 1996).

Here, "collective identity" is in a sense, the "we-awareness consciousness" or a "sense of belonging." This collective identity is expressed through inscriptions and cultural symbols which reflect the attitudes, beliefs, feelings, actions, language, and phrasing of the people (Castile & Kuhner 1981; DeVos 1995).

Among African-Americans, they use terms such as "brother," "sister," "family," and "brethren," to express a feeling of fellowship. In this fictive kinship,

African-Americans who pretend to be Caucasian are targeted with contempt. What does it specifically mean to "pretend to be a Caucasian?"

One of the strategies of African-Americans is "linguistic and cultural integration." They try hard to imitate the behavior and speech of Caucasians because in educational and economic employment environments, abandoning the reference frame of African-Americans, and imitating the reference frame of Caucasians, they will be accepted by white society.

The second coping strategy is to live in both worlds, that of African-Americans and that of Caucasians. In African-American community, they act and talk according to their reference frame, but in the Caucasian's world, such as at school and the workplace, they act and talk according to reference frame of Caucasians.

However, they are aware of ambivalence in the third strategy. In other words, they think about using "proper English" (Caucasian English) to succeed at school and to obtain employment. However, no matter how much they try to speak such English, African style English cannot be totally taken away, and they realize that they are just "pretending to be white." And, in the employment and education environments, they feel that the existing handicap that African-Americans face is not speech and actions but race itself (Obgu 2004).

"Real black" or "spurious black" is evaluated by the standard of fictive kinship. "Real black" is "black like black people," who share experiences, memories, and feelings as African-Americans, and "our friends." On the other hand, "spurious black" are "those people" who abandon "black-like characteristics," betray our black friends, and kowtow to white society.

Fordham and Ogbu (1986) indicated that this fictive kinship is strongly observed in the African-American community and is one factor for the stagnation of academic ability in African-American children. Although slightly off the subject, the problem of mental disorders is introduced here.

In the community of African-Americans, for children to develop high academic ability, obtain a higher educational career, and gain a so-called high-status job, these things are not necessarily positively accepted. The idea that academic work is learning how to play with Caucasians and brings "Caucasian-nizing" beyond the cultural border. It peels away "African-American characteristics" which are tacitly shared among African-Americans as a collective identity, and risks destroying the bonds within the community. Therefore, children of African-Americans tend to pretend that they don't study well or play "the class clown" in order to divert the attention of others from them being "a child who studies hard." And they try to pour their energy into activities which their friends and the African-American community would accept. These conditions are considered to be a factor that suppresses the academic ability of African-American children.

A similar correlation and world view of a fictive kinship are also observed among Zainichi Koreans. Zainichi Koreans have also formed their own collective identity symbolizing camaraderie and bonds between Zainichi Koreans, defending the border against Japanese society, and competing with Japanese society in response to discriminatory and oppressive treatment and the viewpoint of contempt held by Japanese society during the colonial period and after.

For example, in Zainichi Korean society, Koreans refer to each other as "compatriots." Moreover, older persons, even if they do not have a blood relationship, are still called "older brother" or "older sister." Such terms are often heard when many Zainichi Koreans gather together. This custom is still observed even within the younger generation. Within the ethnic organization and groups working on various ethnic activities, the words, "oppa" and "onni" are frequently heard. These mean "older brother" and "older sister" in Korean.

These indicators of ethnic identity of Zainichi Koreans are observed in the fictive kinship and are characterized by Zainichi Koreans objectively confirming each other with such terms as "common ancestor," "same culture," "ethnicity," and "language." In addition, the ethnic identity on which these are based has existed from the beginning, beyond place, time, and culture. It is the concept that the inherited and developed identity will not change during their entire life, but will be passed down to the next generation, and has essentially primitive, inherent, and instinctive characteristics. Such indicators, such as "common ancestor," "same culture," "ethnic," and "language," are in line with the education contents for Zainichi Koreans and North/South Koreans. In other words, viewpoint of the ethnic identity in the education of Zainichi Koreans is considered to have essentially primitive, innate, and instinctive characteristics.

However, since ethnic identity is viewed as primitive, the view of Zainichi Koreans is "an existence which lacks that which should be essentially preserved." However, by this viewpoint, a positive reason to "exist as a Zainichi" is difficult to find. Zainichi Koreans find themselves in an existence that continues to pursue what they lack, without affirming who they really are.

Moreover, doesn't this kind of description of identity have a similar nature as "racism" which asserts that people are decided by their race and ethnicity? In other words, isn't this ethnic education based on the viewpoint derived from determining "true Zainichi Koreans" and "fictive Zainichi Koreans," which is the same logic as the monoracial viewpoint of Japanese society that "the Japanese nation has been established exclusively from the Japanese race with the same language and culture," and "only people of the Japanese race who have a uniform and pure blood line have lived on the Japan peninsula?"

Previously, Hall (1996) expressed cultural identity as a mixed mongrel, which has not been firmly established. In addition, he said that what is called "identity" is in itself only the "tentative positioning," and "as such, each individual story of identity is inscribed in the position of our choosing. It is necessary to live the whole of various identities, while retaining all their particularities as precious."

This identity viewpoint is also applied to Zainichi Korean in many ways. The existence of Zainichi Koreans in Japanese society, which is dominated by monoracial thinking, is also placed in the condition where a "stable" ethnic identity is not possible.

Identity is not something fixed. There are fluid characteristics that can be changed by interaction with other people. If the surrounding people have a positive evaluation of their ethics, Zainichi Koreans also can accept that they are Zainichi Koreans, and carry their own identity. However, if there is a negative evaluation, they will start to have negative self-evaluation and stigma as a Zainichi Korean. Such a dynamic viewpoint of identity is difficult to grasp within the thinking that ethnic identity is primitive, innate, and instinctive. For many Zainichi Koreans, grasping ethnic identity as something real is difficult and vague, and is characterized by the need to fabricate "real facts" due to its abstract nature and non-obviousness.

The primitive, innate, and instinctive viewpoint of ethnic identity which is symbolized by fictive kinship, may be called ethnicity based on "activity logic" which has been accumulated and is comprised based on various vague identities with a specific intention. How Zainichi Koreans live their lives vary, and consequently, how Zainichi Koreans like it should also vary. In the conventional viewpoint that developing ethnic identity is primary, how one lives, what one does to live, and which part he likes about being Zainichi Korean, must consolidated and managed into a fixed image. Instead of pursuing one's identity as a Zainichi Korean in itself, it is important to understand what kind of a Zainichi Korean and what aspects of a Zainichi Korean are sought within one's identity, on the premise of its multi-faceted nature.

However, the previously mentioned fictive kinship relationship as well as the world of Zainichi Koreans has become weaker than before. This is considered to be a result of a decrease in the need for an ethnic community as Zainichi Koreans have achieved a certain degree of stability in their position as the generations progress, which in turn has promoted individualization as well as integration into Japanese society, and "Zainichi Korean" as a common term has become more difficult to encounter.

The view of the fictive kinship world and the discussion on identity of Zainichi Koreans overlap. Zainichi Koreans suffered cultural deprivation under a dominant culture without interruption, and a negative self-consciousness has developed. In that sense, they are ethnically "lacking existence." Consequently, only by fulfilling their ethnic culture by putting forth effort in learning one's own ethnic language, enjoying one's ethnic music and musical instruments, and experiencing one's ethnic food culture, can they become "true ethnics," and overcome conditions of cultural deprivation and negative self-consciousness.

A negative self-impression has been planted in minds of minorities who are placed in an oppressed position by the dominant culture. Free discussion of a positive self-impression and identity is hindered, resulting in the minority internalizing that negative self-impression. Therefore, they are "oppressed persons." The first step to be released from the fetters of the dominant culture and repudiate the inflicted negative nature, is to freely discuss a positive impression as "one's own nature."

By this action, the oppressed persons themselves try to politically correct the negative impression which was forced upon them by the dominant culture, changing it into a positive impression. In other words, they engage in identity politics. However, identity politics as a method to free the oppressed also alienates the diversity within the minority group, by setting "true self-image" (for Zainichi Koreans, the "true Zainichi Korean image").

Kymlicka (1995–1998) called the various rights of minorities demanded by ethnic groups "collective rights," and determined that "many liberal thinkers think that this is characteristically in conflict with personal rights."

In addition, two meanings of these collective rights must be identified. One is the "internal restrictions," which mean the right of a group to restrict the freedom of an individual member, to preserve the solidarity of the group, or in the name of innocence of the culture. The other is "external protections," which mean the right to restrict the economic and/or political authority exercised by the majority in society, in order to protect the resources and system that minority group depends on. In addition, Kymlicka determined "external protections" do not necessarily contradict freedom of individuals, but "internal restrictions" may.

In other words, "external protections" can play a role in ensuring "individual freedom," as a defense measure against oppression received from the dominant society for members of the minority group. However, they may also function to oppress various individual freedoms in the group because they are implemented through "innocence" of the minority group, in contrast to "internal restrictions."

Regarding the concept of Zainichi Koreans, Takeda (1986) stated that especially during the youth of the second generation (in other words, corresponding to the youth of Mr. D) as described in the works of Kim Hak Young, "there are only 'two choices,' that is, a life 'integrated into' Japanese society, or a life dedicated to the integration and establishment of one's homeland as 'a communist.' The important idea is that the <ethnicity> concept for) Zainichi> boils down to the form which ultimately forces a decision between 'accept it or not.'"

The condition of the ethnic organization that Mr. D was involved with, and the generation of his day, was that of "ultimately accept it or not." Zainichi Koreans externally faced various forms of oppression in Japanese society, while the ethnic community served to internally oppress the <individual>. Mr. D was caught in the middle.

5.13 Clinical bias

Finally, "clinical bias" is discussed here.

Kurokawa (2006), quoting from M. Karno, (1966), reasoned on a study that discussed the treatment experience of Mexican-Americans and the relationship between ethnicity, the healer, and the patient. Patients who were minorities were not given sufficient opportunity to receive treatment, and discontinuation of medical care and recurrence were more frequent, and there was a tendency of alienation even by the medical staff (referred to as "therapeutic failure"). These factors were analyzed. A lack of consideration of ethnicity on the healer side, the conventional interview of clinical history, the method of medical care, etc. tended to lead to a neglecting of social and cultural context.

This "clinical bias" is one problem in the medical care and counseling of minorities. Clinical bias is a distortion of clinical judgment and attitude which occurs by the stereotypical viewpoint of counselors toward the minority group with which the patient is affiliated (Wisch & Mahalik 1999; Kodama, et al. 2012). This term especially shows distortion which occurs by the medical staff and counselors as a result of their discriminatory reaction toward minorities. (Lopez, 1989; Kodama, et al. 2012) In addition, Corey and Corey (1998) and Matsutaka (2014) state that separating the values held by assistance workers from their professional relationship is considered almost impossible. It is important for the assistance workers to understand their own values and not force these onto the patient.

As previously considered, contempt and discrimination toward Zainichi Koreans are deeply rooted in Japanese society. Medical staff and counselors are no exception. What if a Zainichi Korean needs support and visits a place where everyone has a negative view of his existence?

What if medical staff and counselors do not recognize this, although the condition of Zainichi Koreans in Japanese society plays a large role in the background of mental disorders? In addition, what if the staff shows contempt and discrimination? The Zainichi Korean may pretend to be an ordinary patient, hiding the fact that he/she is Zainichi Korean in front of the medical staff and counselor. In such a case, essential treatment to improve the disease may not sought, and the medical care and counseling will result in "violence" rather than "saving" for the patient. This is not limited to Zainichi Koreans however. Minorities are people whose access to support to alleviate or eliminate their pain is difficult to guarantee.

6 Establishment of a mental health system for Zainichi Koreans

As described in Kymlicka's "external protections" and "internal restrictions," the issues surrounding "Zainichi" must be considered by separating "issues involving Japanese society and 'Zainichi' society" and the "internal issues of a 'Zainichi.'" "Issues involving Japanese society and 'Zainichi' society" include the view of contempt and discriminatory treatment shown to "Zainichi" that even remains today. "Internal issues of a 'Zainichi'" should also be divided into the consideration of the person's "private sphere" and "public sphere." The private sphere includes family issues within "Zainichi" society, such as the Confucian view on the value of the patriarch within a "Zainichi" household. Issues in the public sphere include problems related to ethnic activities of the "Zainichi," activities within the "Zainichi" community establishment, and empowerment activities of the "Zainichi." Here, I would like to focus on problems in the public sphere, within the internal issues of a "Zainichi."

I personally experienced this when I was young. I used to engage in activities at a "Zainichi" youth organization. At the time, many "Zainichi" children who went to Japanese school were delinquent and suffered from "low academic ability." There is very little data on the academic ability of "Zainichi," but in the statistics of junior high schools in Y city, Osaka prefecture, the rate of high scores, middle scores, and low scores among Japanese students were approximately 30% each. However, among "Zainichi" students, the results were 10%, 25%, and 65%, respectively. Within this, there are various backgrounds, such as lack of future educational prospects due to discrimination or family environment.

At one conference of the organization, I proposed the need for approaches to promote academic ability, although transmitting ethnic culture, such as ethnic music and dance, is also needed. A heated discussion regarding the presentation ensued, and the leader of the organization said, "ensuring academic ability is not within the range of ethnic education." Almost everyone agreed and I was isolated. But I persisted, saying "approaches to promote academic ability are needed," and the comment came out, "That kind of thinking is no good. Quit being a Korean!"

In other words, "ensuring academic ability" is individualism and based on the merit system. "We value the promoting fellowship and developing connections as an ethnic group." Many "Zainichi" who acquire academic ability, establish

DOI: 10.4324/9781003177050-6

an academic career, and gain stable work leave the "Zainichi" community and become immersed in Japanese society, don't they? I'm sure many of them would have liked to say that.

A woman in the organization was engaged in its activities. She always treated me, a newcomer, nicely, and taught me many things which I never knew. However, it seemed that she was also suffering from a lack of confidence in herself. Then she decided to go to South Korea for a year. She said at her send-off party, "I will become stronger and come back." However, I was thinking. "Why don't you just stay where you are? Isn't that your appeal?"

She finished studying at South Korea, and then came back. Just happened to be there when someone said, "Quit being a Korean!"

After the comment of "Quit being a Korean!" among the participants of the heated discussion on "ethnic education vs. ensuring academic ability," she spoke. I thought she would criticize the person who said "quit." I was wrong. Instead, she blamed me saying "why do you force this person to make such a statement?" Honestly, I was speechless. I thought, "Oh, so this is what she meant when she said she would become stronger and come back."

Sorry about talking about a depressing reproach that happened a long time ago, but at the time, this was a symbolic event demonstrating how "violence" could be carried out depending on how ethnic identity is used.

In "Zainichi" activities, ethnic identity aims to be described as having "strength," "cheerfulness," and "monolithic robustness." In such a world, "ambiguity" and "chaotic conditions" tended to be negatively evaluated. But against this trend, "Zainichi" youth crossed the Sea of Genkai and the Sea of Japan seeking to establish and confirm a clear and firm identity.

Someone may ask, "What's wrong with seeking a strong and clear identity?" In itself, there is nothing wrong. However, people who seek "a strong and clear identity" often tend to demand the same of others. And, in many cases, they do not condone ambiguity, chaotic conditions, or vulnerability. For those who are required to have "a strong and clear identity," this can turn into oppression.

What if "Zainichi" activities were "activities without any complaints?" Actually, I knew some of Mr. K's friends introduced in Chapter 2. "I wish they were still alive. I wish I could have seen them again while they were still alive. Shouldn't "Zainichi" pursue more activities that share "weakness," "darkness" and "fragility"?

Finally, this book concludes with a presentation of approaches which focus on the mental health of Zainichi, as "activities of Zainichi to share weakness, darkness and fragility."

6.1 Mental health peer support for Zainichi Koreans

"Peer support" is "support provided by a person in a similar position." Generally, as minority characteristics of a problem increase, the more a person suffers "unspeakable" anxiety. At such a time, peer support is considered to provide great strength to solve problems (Nobuta, 1999).

This may not apply only to "Zainichi." Each person in various positions have their original suffering – women have theirs, men have theirs, and sexual minorities have their own. Each person needs his own strategy to live as he feels fit. Peer support activities for people who are "Zainichi" and in various positions are needed in order for them to gather and talk to each other.

6.2 "Inochi no Denwa (telephone counseling service)" for Zainichi

In Japanese society, the national government, local government, and private organizations operate "Inochi no Denwa (telephone counseling service)." However, even though there are many consultation services in Japanese society, most do not necessarily satisfy the specific needs and anxieties of "Zainichi." An "Inochi no Denwa" (or e-mail, etc.) that specifically targets "Zainichi" is needed.

6.3 Association of bereaved family members of Zainichi suicide victims

As previously shown, the mortality rate of persons with North/South Korean nationality in Japan (or "Zainichi" who have roots in the Korean peninsula) due to suicide is high. As a result, there are many bereaved families of suicide victims and people who have lost friends and acquaintances due to suicide. While Japanese society has associations to support bereaved families of suicide victims, an association for bereaved families of "Zainichi" suicide victims, or a place to provide grief care for persons who have lost friends and acquaintances due to suicide, is needed.

6.4 Education and training activities to increase the number of Zainichi-friendly psychiatrists and support staff

"Clinical bias" is one problem in medical care and counseling for minorities. It is a distortion of clinical judgment and attitude which occurs by stereotypical viewpoint of physicians, counselors, or various support staff members toward the minority group with which the patient is affiliated (Wisch & Mahalik, 1999, Kodama, et al. 2012).

Contempt and discrimination toward "Zainichi" are deeply rooted in Japanese society. Medical staff, counselors, and support staff are no exception. What if a "Zainichi" needs support and visits an agency where everyone has a negative view of his existence? When such happens, the medical care and counseling will result in "violence" rather than "saving." Training of "Zainichi" friendly physicians, counselors, and support staff who understand the conditions of "Zainichi" and their mental health issues is urgent.

6.5 Training of human resources who can practice various approaches

Education and training activities cannot be realized without human resources to facilitate and coordinate approaches 1) to 4), who can provide peer support, handle "inochi no denwa," and support associations for bereaved families of suicide victims. Approaches that utilize training programs and certification systems already established in Japanese society and their application to "Zainichi," and the development of original methods targeting "Zainichi," are needed.

Conclusion

Sociocultural factors related to Zainichi Koreans with mental disorders have been discussed. Like Mr. Youji Kurokawa, I have no intention to generalize the four interview cases into the disposition of Zainichi Koreans or specialize them.

On the other hand, it is also true that the sociocultural factors related to Zainichi Koreans because of who they are uniquely affect the onset and modality of mental disorders.

Zainichi Koreans do not differ from Japanese in racial characteristics that can be externally identified, and they are absorbed into Japanese society culturally as well. Factors related to the onset of mental disorders in this minority group are difficult to visually recognize. Zainichi Koreans do not receive discriminatory treatment because of their cultural differences, but simply because they are Zainichi Korean.

Consequently, in order to identify the psychiatric issues faced by these people, not only should "a different culture" or "multiple cultures" be considered, but another viewpoint is also needed, isn't it? This means power relationship issues, such as discrimination and being discriminated against, or oppression and being oppressed, should be considered. With only the viewpoint of "a different culture," or "multiple cultures," these power relationship issues may be overlooked. Consequently, an actual image of the issue of mental disorders in minorities cannot be obtained.

With the increase in Zainichi foreigners, mental stress and mental disorders of "newcomer foreigners" has attracted attention. Most experiences by newcomer foreigners are also problems faced by Zainichi Koreans both now and in the past. Both groups have historical, cultural, and social originality and commonality. In that sense, these newcomer foreigners can be called "second or third Zainichi Koreans." The experience of Zainichi Koreans is not just a problem of the past, but a problem of today.

I have been interested in the mental disorders, and the relationship between Zainichi Koreans and mental disorders. A long time ago, when the author was young and living in a Zainichi Korean residential area, he heard that "a relatively high rate of Zainichi Koreans experience mental disorder due to their life conditions," and the number of patients at treatment agencies for alcoholism in

DOI: 10.4324/9781003177050-7

southern Osaka who are Zainichi Korean is high. However, most of these stories were only "rumors."

"Mental disorder" in itself tends to carry a stigma. In addition, the existence of Zainichi Koreans is one of discrimination and contempt in Japanese society. Easily connecting the issue of mental disorders with Zainichi Koreans is thought to encourage discrimination and contempt. Still, I wanted to pursue this issue. Since Zainichi Koreans with mental disorders exist outside of Japanese society and on the fringes of "Zainichi Korean society," he wondered if the history, position, experiences, and memory of Zainichi Koreans is concentrated in such existence.

After listening to the history of the four people, I felt this was the epic story of Zainichi Koreans which continued from the first generation to the second and then to the generation after that. And so, I wanted to question Japanese society and Zainichi society about the stories of these four people. He hopes to continue listening to "those without voice" and look intently at the "invisible form" of Zainichi Koreans and continue in this work.

References

Ainu Policy Promotion Office, General Affairs Division, Hokkaido Environment and Life Department, 1998 Understanding the Ainu People.

Akiyama, Kazufumi, Saitou, Jun, 2006 "Stress and Psychiatric Disorders" in Dokkyo Journal of Medical Sciences 33(3), pp. 207–212, Dokkyo Medical University.

American Psychiatric Association, 2013 Diagnostic and Statistical Manual of Mental Disorders: Fifth Edition (DSM-5), American Psychiatric Publishing.

Anderson, Benedict, 1983 Imagined Communities: Reflection on the Origin and Spread of Nationalism, Verso.

Barth, Frederik, 1969 "Introduction" in Barth, Frederik (ed.), Ethnic Group and Boundaries: The Social Organization of Culture Difference, Little Brown and Company

Berry, John W., 2005 "Acculturation: Living Successfully in Two Cultures" in International Journal of Intercultural Relations 29, pp. 697–712.

Berry, John W., 2008 "Globalization and Acculturation" in International Journal of Intercultural Relations 32, pp. 328–336.

Boardman, Jason S., Finch, Brian Karl, Ellison, Christopher G., David, R., 2001 "Neighborhood Disadvantage, Stress, and Drug Use Among Adults" in Journal of Health and Social Behavior 42, pp. 151–165.

Bogardus, Emory S., 1933 "A Social Distance Scale" in Sociology and Social Research 17, pp. 265–271.

Bombay, Amy et al., 2014 The Intergenerational Effects of Indian Residential Schools: Implications for the Concept of Historical Trauma, SAGE.

Bombay, Amy, 2014, Intergenerational Trauma:Convergence of Multiple Processes among First Nations peoples in Canada. https://www.researchgate.net/profile/Amy_Bombay/publication/242778748_Intergenerational_Trauma/links/0c960527 6e0d7a67e8000000/Intergenerational-Trauma.pdf

Bratter, Jenifer L., Eschbach, Karl, 2005 "Race/Ethnic Differences in Nonspecific Psychological Distress: Evidence from the National Health Interview Survey" in Social Science Quarterly 86(3), pp. 620–644.

Breslau, J, Aguilar-Gaxiola, S, Kendler, KS, Su, M, Williams, D, Kessler, RC., 2006 "Specifying Race-Ethnic Differences in Risk for Psychiatric Disorder in a USA National Sample" in Psychological Medicine 36(1), pp. 57–68.

Brown, Rupert, 2010 Prejudice: Its Social Psychology (Second Edition), Wiley-Blackwell.

Burnam, M. Audrey, Hough, Richard L., Karno, Marvin, Escobar, Javier I., Telles, Cynthia A., 1987. "Acculturation and Lifetime Prevalence of Psychiatric Disorders Among Mexican Americans in Los Angeles" in Journal of Health and Social Behavior 28, pp. 89–102.

Butler, J., 1990 Gender Trouble: Feminism and the Subversion of Identity, Routledge.

Cabinet Office Task Force on Suicide Prevention, The Community Safety Planning Division of the Community Safety Bureau of the National Police Agency, 2015 The Referential Diagram of Suicides Based on the Suicide Statistics.

Cantor-Graae, E., Selten, J.P., 2005 "Schizophrenia and Migration: A Meta-Analysis and Review" in The American Journal of Psychiatry 162(1), pp. 12–24.

Castile, G.P., Kushner, G., 1981 Persistent Peoples: Cultural Enclaves in Perspective, University of Arizona Press.

Chizuko, Ueno, 1996, "Complex Discrimination Theory" in Shun Inoue, Chizuko Ueno, Masachi Osawa, Munesuke Mita and Shunya Yoshimi, "Iwanami Lecture Contemporary Sociology 15 Sociology of Discrimination and Coexistence" Iwanami Shoten, 203–232.

Cikap, Mieko, 1991 The Blessing of the Wind, Ochanomizu Shobo.

Cockerham, William C., 2016 Sociology of Mental Disorder (Ninth edition), Routledge.

Cohen, Abner, 1974 "Introduction: The Lesson of Ethnicity" in Cohen, Abner (ed.), Urban Ethnicity, Tavistock Publications.

Cohen, Ronald, 1978 "Ethnicity: Problem and Focus in Anthropology", Annual Review of Anthropology.

Committee on the Protection of Rights of Koreans in Japan, 1996 White Paper of the Human Rights of Korean Residents in Japan.

Corey, M.S., Corey, G., 1998 Becoming a Helper, Brooks/Cole Publishing Company.

De Vos, G.A. 1975 "Ethnic Pluralism: Conflict and Accommodation" in De Vos, G & Romanucci-Ross, L. (eds.), Ethnic Identity: Cultural Continuities and Change.

DeVos, G.A., 1992 Social Cohesion and Alienation: Minorities in the United States and Japan, Westview Press.

DeVos, G.A., 1995 "Ethnic Pluralism: Conflicts and Accommodation" in L. Romanucci-Ross & G. A. DeVos (Eds.), Ethnic Identity: Creation, Conflict, and Accommodation, Altimira Press, pp. 15–41.

DeVos, G.A., Suarez-Orozco, Marcelo, 1990 Status Inequality: The Self in Culture, Sage Publication.

Dovidio, John F., Gaertner, Samuel L., 2004 "Aversive Racism, Advances" in Experimental Social Psychology 36, pp. 1–52.

Duran, B., Sanders, M., Skipper, B., Waitzkin, H., Malcoe, L.H., Paine, S., et al., 2004 "Prevalence and correlates of mental disorders among Native American women in primary care" in American Journal of Public Health 94(1), pp. 71–77.

Eiji, Oguma, 1995 A Genealogy of Japanese Self-Images, Shinyosha.

Fanon, F., 1951 Peau Noire, Masques Blanc, Seuil.

Fingerhut, L.A., MaKue, D.M., 1992 "Mortality Among Minority Populations in the United States" in American Journal of Public Health 82(8), pp. 1168–1170.

Fordham, Signithia, Ogbu, John. U., 1986 "Black students' School Success: Coping With the "burden of 'acting white'" in Urban Review 18(3), pp. 176–206.

Fordham, Signithia, 1996 Blacked Out: Dilemmas of Race, Identity, and Success at Capital High, University of Chicago Press.

Fujita, Keiichi ed., 1998 What Is "Burakumin?", Aunsha.

Fukuoka, Yasunori, 1993 Japan-resident Koreans: The Identity of the Younger Generation, Chuokoron-Shinsha.

Geertz, Clifford, 1973 The Interpretation of Cultures, Basic Books.

Gitlin, Todd, 1993 "The Rise of 'Identity Politics,'" in Dissent 40 (Spring1993), pp. 172–175.

Goffman, E., 1963 Stigma: Notes on the Management of Spoiled Identity, Simon & Schuster.

Gyeongsig, Seo, 1996 "Beyond Multiculturalism" in Impaction 99, Impact Shuppankai.

Hall, Stuart, 1986 "Gramsci's Relevance for the Study of Race and Culture" in Journal of Communication Inquiry 10(Summer).

Hall, Stuart, 1989 "Ethnicity: Identity and Difference" Edited version of a speech delivered at Hampshire College.

Hall, Stuart, 1990 "Cultural Identity and Diaspora" in Jonathan Rutherford (ed.), Identity: Community, Culture, Difference, Lawrence & Wishart.

Hall, Stuart, 1996 "Critical Dialogues" in Thought 859 translated by Hiroki Ogasawara, Iwanami Shoten.

Halpern, D., 1993 "Minorities and Mental Health" in Social Science & Medicine 36, pp. 597–607.

Harima, Katsumi, Ishimaru, Keiichirou, 2010 "Gender Identity Disorder and Suicide" in Japanese Journal of Psychiatric Treatment 25(2), pp. 245–251, Seiwa Shoten.

Harris, K.M., Edlund, M.J., Larson, S., 2005 "Racial and Ethnic Differences in the Mental Health Problems and Use of Mental Health Care" in Medical Care 43(8), pp. 775–784.

Henderson, Kellina C., Sloan, L.R., 2003 "After the Hate: Helping Psychologists Help Victims of Racist Hate Crime" in Clinical Psychology: Science and Practice 10(4), pp. 481–490.

Hechter, Michael, 1974 "The Political Economy of Ethnic Change", American Journal of Sociology 79-5 1976, "Ethnicity and Industrialization: On the Proliferation of the Cultural Division of Labor", Ethnicity 3.

Hidaka, Y., Operario, D., Takenaka, M., Omori, S., Ichikawa, S., Shirasaka, T., 2008 "Attempted Suicide and Associated Risk Factors Among Youth in Urban Japan" in Social Psychiatry and Psychiatric Epidemiology 43(9), pp. 752–757.

Hobsbawm, Eric, 1985 "Introduction: Inventing Traditions" in Hobsbawm, Eric & Ranger, Terence (eds.), The Invention of Tradition, Cambridge UP.

Hobsbawm, Eric, 1990 Nations and Nationalism Since 1780, Cambridge UP.

Husaini, B.A., Sherkat, D.E., Levine, R., Bragg, R., Hoizer, C., Anderson, K., et al., 2002 "Race, gender, and health care service utilization and costs among Medicare elderly with psychiatric diagnoses" in Journal of Aging and Health 14(1), pp. 79–95.

Ikeda, Hiroshi, 1985 Educational Attainment of "Buraku" Youth and Its Cultural Background: Ethnography of a Rural "Buraku" Community and Lifestyle of Youth, Bulletin of The Faculty of Human Sciences, Osaka University 11.

Ikeda, Hiroshi, 1989 "Self-Concept and Achievement" in Research for Emancipatory Education 2 edited by Research Institute for Emancipatory Education.

Im, Mutaeg, 2011 The History of the Alliance of Korean Youths from 1960s to 1980s - The Racial Movement and Identity of the Second Generation of Korean Residents in Japan, Shinkansha.

Immigration Bureau, Ministry of Justice, 1949 Immigration Control.

Isaacs, Harold R. 1975, "Basic Group Identity: The Idol of the Tribe" in Glazer, N. & Moynihan, D. P. (eds.) Ethnicity: Theory and Experience, Harvard UP.

Isajiw, Wsevolod W., 1974 "Definition of Ethnicity", Ethnicity 1–2.

Itou Abito et al., Cyclopedia of Korea under the supervision, Heibonsha.1986.

Izawa, Yasuki (Taeyoung, Kim), Korean Youth Union in Japan, 2013 Survey Report on Hate Speech and Perceptions of History.

Izawa, Yasuki (Taeyoung, Kim), Korean Youth Union in Japan, 2015 The Investigation Report on the Actual State of Hate Speech against Korean Residents in Japan and Discrimination against Korean Youth in Japan Regarding Internet Use.

Jackson, Pamela Braboy., 1997 "Role Occupancy and Minority Mental Health" in Journal of Health and Social Behavior 38, pp. 237–255.

Jung, Yeonghae, 1994 "Toward Open Families – The Complex Identity and Right to Self-Determination" in The Annual Report of the Women's Studies 15.

Jung, Yeonghae, 1996 "Beyond the Identity" in Sociology of Discrimination and Coexistence, Iwanami Shoten.

Jun, Kamata, 2009 Native American - Current of Indigenous Communities, Iwanami Shoten.

Kang, Cheol ed., 2002. The General History Chart of Korean Residents in Japan, Yuzankaku.

Kang, Sangjung, 1995 "Ethnicity and Universal Principles" in The Asahi Shinbun, November 16, 1995.

Karno, M., 1966 "The Enigma of Ethnicity in a Psychiatric Clinic" in Arch. Gen. Psychiat. 14, pp. 516–520.

Kashiwazaki, Chikako, 2007 "Being a 'Korean' without South or North Korean Nationality - The Display of Korean Identity of Those with Japanese Nationality" in North America, East Asia, Central Asia- Koreans as Diaspora compiled under the supervision of Gojeon, Hyeseong, translated by Chikako Kashiwazaki, Shinkansha, pp. 195–228.

Kasuga, Takehiko, 2006 Schizophrenia, Shufunotomo.

Katou, Masaaki ed., 2001 Encyclopedia of Psychiatry - Reduced-size edition, Koubundou.

Katou, Satoshi, Kanba, Shigenobu, Nakatani, Youji, Takeda, Masatoshi, Kashima, Haruo, Kano, Rikihachirou, Ichikawa, Hironobu ed., 2011 Encyclopedia of Contemporary Psychiatry, Koubundou.

Keira, Mitsunori, 1997 "Discrimination and Coexistence Regarding the Ainu" in Toward Coexistence (Lecture: The Sociology of Discrimination, 4), Koubundou.

Kessler, Ronald C., Neighbors, Harold W., 1986. "A New Perspective on the Relationships between Race, Social Class, and Psychological Distress" in Journal of Health and Social Behavior 27, pp. 107–115.

Kessler, Ronald C., Mickelson, Kristin D., Williams, David R., 1999. "The Prevalence, Distribution, and Mental Health Correlates of Perceived Discrimination in the United States" in Journal of Health and Social Behavior 40, pp. 208–230.

Keyes, Charles F., 1976 "Towards a New Formulation of the Concept of Ethnic Group", Ethnicity 3-3 1981 "The Dialectics of Ethnic Change" in Keyes, Charles F (ed.), Ethnic Change, Washington UP.

Kim, Jangsu, 2001 "The Identity and Psychiatric Disorders of Korean Residents in Japan - Especially About the Zainichi Syndrome" in Masaya Yamashita, Kim, Sunghyo and Mitsuo Higuma (eds.), The Identity of Korean Residents in Japan and Japanese Society - The Opinion on a Tolerant, Multi-Ethnic Society, Akashi Shoten, pp. 76–122.

Kim, Gyeonghae, 1979 The Origin of the Ethnic Education of Korean Residents in Japan - The Document About Hanshin Educational Struggle on April 24, Tabata Shoten.

Kim, Gyeonghae, 1988 The Documents of the Defense Struggle for the Ethnic Education of Korean Residents in Japan, Akashi Shoten.

Kim, Taehong and Lee Insok, 2007, "A Change in Confucian Country, South Korea: Changes in Family Views and Declining Birthrate," International Cultural Studies, No. 11, 119–128.

Taeyoung, Kim, 1999 Beyond Identity Politics – The Ethnicity of Korean Residents in Japan, Akashi Shoten.

Taeyoung, Kim, 2017 Korean Residents in Japan and Psychiatric Disorders - A Life History and Social Environment as the Factors, Koyo Shobo.

Kleinman, Arthur, 1991 Rethinking Psychiatry: from Cultural Category to Personal Experience, Free Press.

Kodama, Kenichi, Shinagawa, Yuka, Tsuruta, Kazumi, Amitani, Ayaka, Iwakiri, Sachiko, Kurita, Tomomi, 2012 "Practice of Dynamic Psychology in a Clinical Setting," in written by Yuuko Okamoto and Kenichi Kodama, (eds.), The New Century of Psychological Research 4 Clinical Psychology, Under the Supervision of Hiromi Fukada, Minerva Shobo.

Kurokawa, Kisyou, 1987 Philosophy of Symbiosis, Tokuma Shoten.

Kurokawa, Youji, 2006 North and South Korean Residents in Japan and Mental Health in Japan, Hihyo-sha.

Kymlicka, Will, 1995 Multicultural Citizenship: A Liberal Theory of Minority Rights, Oxford University Press.

Laveist, Thomas A, Isaac Lydia A eds., 2013 Race, Ethnicity, and Health: A Public Health Reader (Second Edition), John Wiley & Sons.

Lee, Chagsoo, DeVos, George et al., 1982 Koreans in Japan: Ethnic Conflict and Accommodation, University of California Press.

Lee, Gwang-il 1985 "Ethnicity and Modern Society - Attempts on a Political Sociological Approach" in Thought 730.

Lee, Hongjang, 2008 "Through the Life Stories of 'Doubles' between the Zainichi-Chousenjin and the Japanese" in Kyoto Journal of Sociology 16, pp. 75–96.

Lee, Hongjang, 2016 The Ethnic Experience of Being Korean Residents in Japan - For Reconsideration of Communal Nature Based on Individuals, Seikatsushoin.

Lee, Jeonghee, Tomoko Tanaka, 2011 "Implications for Zainichi Korean Research from a Review of Acculturation Attitudes and Cultural Identity in Overseas Immigrants (1): Focusing on a Bidimensional Model of Acculturation and Psychological Variable" in Journal of Humanities and Social Sciences, Published by Graduate School of Humanities and Social Sciences Okayama University 32, pp. 123–137.

Lewin, K., 1948 Resolving Social Conflicts, Harper's.

Lopez, S.R., 1989 "Patient variable Biases in Clinical Judgment: Conceptual Overview and Methodological Considerations in Psychological Bulletin 106, pp. 184–203.

Loue, Sana, Sajatovic, Martha eds., 2010 Determinants of Minority Mental Health and Wellness, Springer.

Matsuda, Motoji, 1996a "Facts and Fictions About Ethnic Groups" in Takuzou Isobe and Masataka Katagiri (eds.), The Society as a Fiction - The Reconstruction of Sociology, Sekaishisosha.

Matsuda, Motoji, 1996b "Two Varying Memories – Stories of the War Related by Korean Atomic Bomb Survivors Forced to Work at Mitsubishi Factories" in Impaction 99, Impact Shuppankai.

Matsutaka, Yuka, 2014 "The Influence That Values of Psychologists Regarding Sexuality Exercises on Their Therapies" in Disorders written by Katsumi Harima and Toshiaki Hirata (eds.), Psychological Support to Sexual Minorities - Understanding Homosexuality and Gender Identity Iwasaki Academic Publisher, pp. 229–237.

Michihiro Okuda, Yasuo Hirota and Junko Tajima (eds.), 1994 Foreign Residents and the Japanese Community, Akashi Shoten.

Ministry of Health, Labour and Welfare, 2009 To Support Suicide - Bereaved Family Members - Guidelines for Those in Charge of Counseling - Support and Care for Those Bereaved by Suicide, 2015 Population Dynamics in Japan - Population Dynamics Statistics Including Foreigners - (FY 2014).

Ministry of Justice, 2016 Concerning the Number of Foreign Residents at the End of 2015.

Minzoku-Kyouiku-Sokusin-Kyougikai, 1995 Ten-year History of Minsokukyo - Providing Ethnic Education for All Compatriots.

Minzoku-Sabetsu-to-Tatakau-Renrakukai, 1992 Providing Ethnic Education in Anti-Discrimination and Human Rights.

Minzokumei-wo-Trimodosu-Kai, 1990 Koreans With Japanese Nationality Who Restore the Names of the Ethnic Group, Akashi Shoten.

Mizuno, Naoki, Mun, Gyeongsu, 2015 Korean Residents in Japan - Their History and Present State, Iwanami Shoten.

Miyaji, Naoko, 2005 Traumatic Medical Anthropology, Misuzu Shobo.

Miyaji, Naoko, 2013 Traumas, Iwanami Shoten.

Moon, Gyonsu, 2005 "Modern History of Jeju Island: Death and Rebirth of the Public Sphere", Shinkansha.

Morooka, Yasuko, 2013 What Is Hate Speech? Iwanami Shoten.

Moto, Yuriko, 2018, "International Development of the Concept of Multiple Discrimination," Buraku Liberation, No. 753, 12–19.

Mun, Gyeongsu, 2005 Korean Modern History, Iwanami Shoten.

Nakajima, Tomoko, 1994 "The Education and the Ethnicity of Korean Residents in Japan: from the Perspective of "Cultural Orientation" and "Social Orientation" in The Japanese Journal of Education Research 61(3).

Nakano, Syuuichirou, 1993 "Refugees from Indochina - Considering Through the Experiences at the Himeji Settlement Promotion Centre" in Syuuichirou Nakano and Koujiro Imazu (eds.), Sociology of Ethnicity Sekaishisosha.

Nariai-niokeru-Zainichi-Korean-no-seikatsusi Goudou-Hensyuuiinkai, 1980 We Have Lived in This Way.

Naroll, Raoul, 1964 "On Ethnic Unit Classification", Current Anthropology 5-4.

National Center of Neurology and Psychiatry, The Working Group on the Recommendation for Revision of the General Principles of Suicide Prevention, 2012 Recommendation for Revision of the General Principles of Suicide Prevention Policy (the final proposal).

Neff, James Alan, Husani, Baoar A., 1987 "Urbanicity, Race, and Psychological Distress" in Journal of Community Psychology 1, pp. 520–36.

Nobuta, Sayoko, 1999, Addition Approach: Another Family Assistance Theory, Igaku-Shoin.

Noguchi, Masayuki, 2008 "Schizophrenia - From the Perspective of Cultural and Social Psychiatry" in Masaaki Matsushita, Satoshi Katou and Shigenobu Kanba (eds.), PSychiatric Dialogue,KOUBUNDOU, pp. 453–472.

Nomura, Giichi, 1996 Living in the Ainu, Sofukan.

Oda, Makoto, 1996a "Intellect of Flexible Wild Nature" in Tamotsu Aoki et al. (eds.), Turning the Neighboring World into a System of Thought. Iwanami Shoten.

Oda, Makoto, 1996b "The Price of Postmodern Anthropology" in Bulletin of the National Museum of Ethnology 1996–21 (4).

Ogasawara, Nobuyuki, 1997 Ainu Discrimination Issues Handbook, Ryokufu Shuppan.

Ogbu, John U., Simons, Herbert D., 1998 "Voluntary and Involuntary Minorities: A Cultural-Ecological Theory of School Performance With Some Implications for Education" in Anthropology & Education Quarterly 29(2), pp. 155–188.

Ogbu, John U., 2004 "Collective Identity and the Burden of "Acting White" in Black History, Community, and Education" in The Urban Review 36(1).

Oohashi, Kazue, 1980 "Cultural Marginality and Clinical Social Pathology" in Hiroshi Iwai and Akira Fukushima (eds.), Modern Clinical Social Pathology, Iwasaki Academic Publisher, pp. 377–391.

Ookoshi, Aiko, 1996 Introducing Feminism, Chikuma Shobo.

Oosakafu-Zainichigaikokujin-Kyouiku-Kenkyuukyougikai, 1997 The Idea of Multicultural Education with a Vision for the 21st Century - The Education of Foreign Residents That Fugaikyo Promotes.

Oosugi, Takashi, 1999 Creoleness and Alterity, Iwanami Shoten.

Oota, Junichi, 1996 Osaka Uchinanchu, Brain Center.

Oota, Yosinobu, 1992 "Objectification of Culture" in The Japanese Journal of Ethnology 57(3).

Orihara, Hiroshi, 1969 Human and Learning in Time of Crisis - The Marginal Man Theory and the Transformation of the Image of Weber, Mirai-sha.

Ozawa, Yuusaku, 1973 The Educational Theory of Korean Residents in Japan - History, Akishobo.

Pak, Gyeongsig, 1989 After the Liberation - The History of the Movement of Korean Residents in Japan, San-Ichi Publishing.

Pak, Shàngdeug, 1980 The Ethnic Education of Korean Residents in Japan, Ariesu Shobo.

Park, Robert E., 1928 "Human Migration and the Marginal Man" in The American Journal of Sociology 33(6), pp. 881–893.

Rekishi-Kyoukasyo Zainichi-Korean-no-Rekishi hensyuu-Iinkai (ed.), 2013 The History Textbook - The History of Korean Residents in Japan (The second edit.), Akashi Shoten.

Portes, Alejandro, 1981, "Modes of structural incorporation and present theories of labor immigrations" in Kritz MM, Keely CB, Tomasi SM, (eds), Global trends in migration. CMS Press, 279–297.

Riesman, David, 1953–1954 "Some Observation on Intellectual Freedom", The American Scholar 23-1.

Royce, Anya, 1982 "Neither Christian nor Jewish" in Ethnic Identity: Strategies of Diversity, Indiana UP.

Sakamoto, Shinji, Tanno, Yoshihiko, Oono, Yutaka (eds.), 2005 Clinical Psychology of Depression, University of Tokyo Press.

Schiller Nina G.,2005, Long-Distance Nationalism,Encyclopedia of diasporas 2005 Edition. https://link.springer.com/referenceworkentry/10.1007%2F978-0-387299044_ 59#:~:text=Definition,see%20as%20their%20ancestral%20home.

Sekine, Masami, 1994 The Political Sociology of Ethnicity, The University of Nagoya Press.

Segal, Lynne, 1989 Is the Future Female? Translated by Motoko Oda, Keiso Shobo.

Selye, H., 1956 The Stress of Life (The second edit.), McGraw-Hill Education.

Shils, Edward, 1957 "Primordial, Personal, Sacred, and Civil Ties", *British Journal of Sociology* 8, pp. 130–145

Shinozaki, Heiji, 1955 The Movement of Korean Residents in Japan, Reibunsha.

Smith, Anthony D., 1989 "The Origins of Nations", Ethnic and Racial Studies 12-3.

Sollors, Werner, 1989 "Introduction: The Invention of Ethnicity" in Sollors, Werner (ed.) The Invention of Ethnicity, Oxford UP.

Stepleman, L.S., Wright, D.E., Bottonari, K.A., 2010 "Socioeconomic Status: Risk and Resilience" in S. Loue, M. Sajatovic (Eds.), Determinants of Minority Mental Health and Wellness, Springer, pp. 273–302.

Stonequist, E.V., 1937 The Marginal Man: A Study in Personality and Culture Conflict, Charles Scribner's Sons.

Sugi, Yasusaburou, Tatai, Kichinosuke, Fujii, Naoharu, Takemiya, Takashi (trans), 1988 The Stress of Life, Hosei University Press.

Tadashi, Kaizawa, 1972 "Going on an Excursion with One Broiled Fish" in Ushio 150.

Takatsuki-Mukuge-no-kai, 1984 Korean Residents in Takatsuki - The Investigation Report on the Actual State - Life, Environment, Labor, Health and Education.

Takatsuki-Mukuge-no-kai, 1992 It is interesting because it is an Ethnic Group - The Commemorative Publication to Mark the 20th Anniversary of the Foundation of Takatsuki-Mukuge-no-kai.

Takatsuki-Omoni-no-kai, 1997 Omoni 50.

Takatsukisi-Kyouiku-Iinkai, 1996 Goals and Plans for the Educational Activities of Korean Residents in Japan in FY 1996.

Takatsukisi-Zainichigaikokujin-Kyouiku-Kenkyuu-Kyougikai, 1997 Chindarure 13.

Takayama, Mami, 2012 The Current State of "Discrimination, Hatred and Dependence" in The African-American Community–Living With an African-American Family in Chicago, Akishobo.

Tanimoto, Emi, 2012 Moral Harassment Explained by a Counselor - What You Can Do to Take Your Life Back, Shobunsha.

Takeda, Seiji, 1986 "The Protyle of Suffering" in The Collection of the Works of Kim Hak Young, Sakuhinsha.

Takezawa, Yasuko, 1994 The Transformation of Japanese American Ethnicity: The Effects of Internment and Redress, University of Tokyo Press.

Tomoko, Nakajima, 1991 "The Debate and Issues Concerning Multicultural Education" in The Seizan Gakuho 39, Kyoto Seizan College.

Tomiyama, Ichirou, 1990 "Okinawajin" in Modern Japanese Society, Nihon Keizai Hyouronsha.

Tsujiuchi, Makoto, 1994 "Historical Context of Multiculturalism and the American Political Culture" in Thought 843.

van den Berghe, P.L., 1978 "Race and Ethnicity: A Sociological Perspective", Ethnic and Racial Studies 1-4.

Wagatsuma, Hiroshi, Yoneyama, Toshinao, 1967 Structure of Prejudice - Japanese View of Race, NHK Publishing.

World Health Organization (WHO), 2014 Preventing Suicide: a global imperative.

Williams, D.R., Harris-Reid, M., 1999 "Race and Mental Health: Emerging Patterns and Promising Approaches" in A.V. Horowitz, T.L. Scheid (Eds.), A Handbook for the Study of Mental Health: Social Contexts, Theories, and Systems, Cambridge University Press, pp. 295–314.

Wisch, A.F., Mahalik, J.R., 1999 "Male Therapists' Clinical Bias: Influence of Client Gender Roles and Therapist Gender Role Conflict" in Journal of Counseling Psychology 46, pp. 51–60.

Xie, Yu & Gough, Margaret(2011). Ethnic Enclaves and the Earnings of Immigrants, Demography, vol.48, pages1293–1315. https://www.ncbi.nlm.nih.gov/pmc/articles/PMC3226926/#R31

Yang, Taeho, 1996 The Handbook of Korean Residents in Japan, Ryokufu Shuppan.

Yang, Taeho, Yamada, Takao, 2014 New Handbook of South and North Korean Residents in Japan, Ryokufu Shuppan.

Yang, Yeonghu, 1985 "Educational Issues of Children from Korean Residents in Japan" in Lecture: Discrimination and Human Rights 4 Ethnic Groups, Yuzankaku.

Yang, Yongja, 1985, "Booklet of Working Friends", edited by the Joint Editorial Committee, "Rejection of Fingerprints!-Discrimination/division/management out-of-law system" Shinchiheisya.

Yoshirou, Nabeshima, 1993 "Burakumin Minority and Their Educational Attainment - Using J.U. Ogbu's Anthropological Approach as a Lead" in Studies of Educational Sociology 52, The Japan Society of Educational Sociology, Toyokan Publishing, pp. 208–231.

Yun, Geoncha, 1987 Coexistence With Heterogeneousness, Iwanami Shoten.

Index

Note: **Bold** folios indicate tables and *italics* indicate figures in the text.

For Product Safety Concerns and Information please contact our EU
representative GPSR@taylorandfrancis.com
Taylor & Francis Verlag GmbH, Kaufingerstraße 24, 80331 München, Germany

www.ingramcontent.com/pod-product-compliance
Lightning Source LLC
Chambersburg PA
CBHW060320220326
41598CB00027B/4379